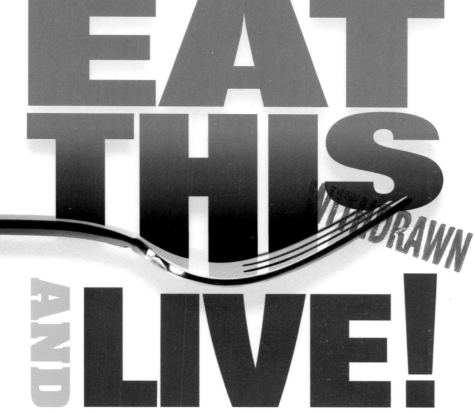

EAT THIS AND LIVE!

DON COLBERT, MD

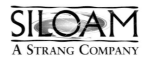

SILOAM
A STRANG COMPANY

Most Strang Communications Book Group products are available at special quantity discounts for bulk purchase for sales promotions, premiums, fund-raising, and educational needs. For details, write Strang Communications Book Group, 600 Rinehart Road, Lake Mary, Florida 32746, or telephone (407) 333-0600.

Eat This and Live! by Don Colbert, MD
Published by Siloam, A Strang Company
600 Rinehart Road, Lake Mary, Florida 32746
www.strangbookgroup.com

Unless otherwise noted, all Scripture quotations are from the New King James Version of the Bible. Copyright © 1979, 1980, 1982 by Thomas Nelson, Inc., publishers. Used by permission.

Scripture quotations marked KJV are from the King James Version of the Bible.

Scripture quotations marked NIV are from the Holy Bible, New International Version. Copyright © 1973, 1978, 1984, International Bible Society. Used by permission.

Scripture quotations marked NLT are from the Holy Bible, New Living Translation, copyright © 1996, 2004. Used by permission of Tyndale House Publishers, Inc., Wheaton, IL 60189. All rights reserved.

Design Director: Bill Johnson
Cover design by Justin Evans; Interior design by Karen Grindley, Jeanne Logue, Debbie Marrie

Library of Congress Cataloging-in-Publication Data

Colbert, Don.
 Eat this and live / Don Colbert.
     p. cm.
 Includes bibliographical references and index.
 ISBN 978-1-59979-519-5
 1. Nutrition. 2. Medicine, Popular. 3. Food--Religious aspects. I.
Title.
 RA784.C5666 2009
 613.2--dc22
                              2008042054

Available as an e-book from Barnes & Noble.

People and incidents in this book are composites created by the author from his experiences as a medical doctor. Names and details of the stories have been changed, and any similarity between the names and stories of individuals described in this book to individuals known to readers is purely coincidental.

Mention of specific companies, organizations, or authorities in this book does not imply their endorsement of this book, nor does it imply the publisher's endorsement of the above. While the author has made every effort to provide accurate telephone numbers and Internet addresses at the time of publication, neither the publisher nor the author assumes any responsibility for errors or for changes that occur after publication.

The nutrition facts for restaurants and brand-name products mentioned in this book were made public by their companies. For companies who do not provide complete nutrition information to the public, the estimates for their products were obtained from www.healthydiningfinder.com and www.thedailyplate .com. This book should not be regarded as a substitute for professional medical treatment, and the author, publisher, manufacturers, or distributors cannot accept legal responsibility for any problem arising out of the use of or experimentation with the methods described.

10 11 12 13 14 — 11 10 9 8 7
Printed in the United States of America

THIS BOOK IS DEDICATED TO OUR CHILDREN.

This is the first generation in history that is not expected to live as long as their parents. As parents we should be examples of health and healthy eating for our children. We need to love our children enough to teach them which foods to eat and which to avoid. We also need to keep junk food and sugary foods out of the house. Hosea 4:6 says, "My people are destroyed for lack of knowledge"—not a lack of prayer, a lack of faith, or a lack of love, but a lack of knowledge. I pray that *Eat This and Live!* arms you and your family with the knowledge you need to make this generation the healthiest generation!

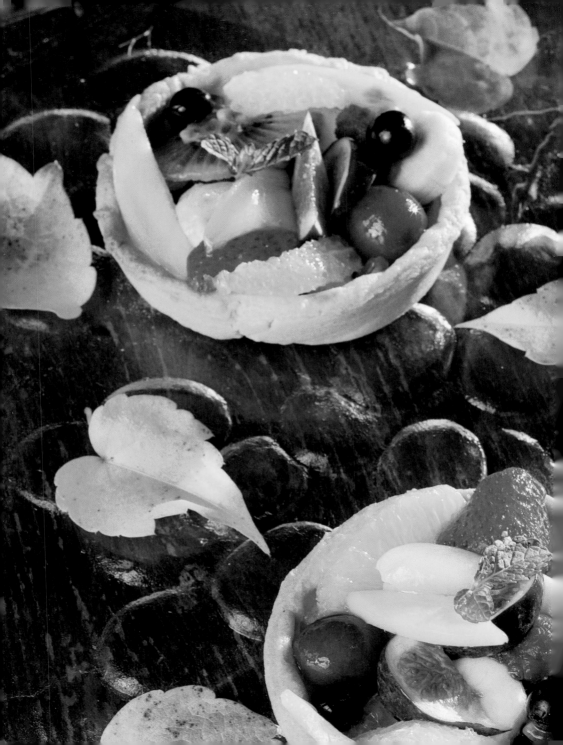

CONTENTS

INTRODUCTION

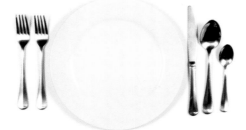

WHEN I WROTE *The Seven Pillars of Health,* I introduced people to the seven basic pillars of a healthy lifestyle. I believe that by living out the seven principles I shared in that book, anyone can become stronger, healthier, more energetic, younger looking, wiser, smarter, and more disease resistant.

As a medical doctor who is board certified in family practice and anti-aging, I have dedicated my life to helping people become healthy. Because I have spent more than twenty years treating patients, the advice I give in my books is based on my years of experience with real problems and real people.

One area of health that I commonly address when treating my patients is their diet. Why? Because research has shown us over and over again that too many Americans are eating their way to an early grave! The key is to know what foods to eat heartily, what foods to eat in moderation, and what foods to avoid. Wouldn't it be great if there were a road map to help you navigate through the often-treacherous territory of healthy food choices? That is exactly what you hold in your hands.

The first several chapters of this book come from Pillar 3 of *The Seven Pillars of Health,* where I lay the groundwork to help you obtain a deeper understanding of why some foods are healthy ("living") and some are unhealthy ("dead"). In the remaining chapters I've removed the guesswork by giving you my picks of the healthiest food items in your grocery store and many popular fast-food and casual-dining restaurants. I've also provided you with tips for storing and preparing food in the healthiest ways possible, along with tips for getting your children to eat more healthily too. As a result, this is an extremely practical guidebook that teaches you how to adopt a dietary lifestyle that is maintainable for years to come. My goal is not to make eating a chore or to make more work on your part, but to enable you to exchange old habits for new ones.

You'll notice that the title of this book is not *Don't Eat This and Live.* Far from being a "don't, can't, shouldn't" book, *Eat This and Live!* is designed to liberate you and help you make choices that bring you freedom in every area of life. It's not about what you are *giving up*; it's about what you are *adding* to your life. It's not about what you *can't* do; it's about what you *can* do to start looking and feeling better than ever.

In the Old Testament, God gave the Israelites a choice. He said, "I have set before you life and death, blessing and cursing; therefore, choose life, that both you and your descendants may live" (Deut. 30:19). That was thousands of years ago, but I believe we still have a life-and-death choice before us today. We can choose to eat unhealthy foods that bring about degeneration and accelerate the aging process, or we can choose to eat living foods that help protect our bodies from disease and give us more vitality.

Imagine yourself standing at a crossroads. In the middle is a road sign with two arrows pointing in opposite directions. It tells you that if you follow one arrow, you can "eat this and die," but if you follow the other arrow, you can "eat this and live." My hope is that you will choose the path that leads to life.

And by life, I don't mean mere survival. Unlike some authors of books about nutrition, I believe that God has given us food, like life, to *enjoy*. I have written *Eat This and Live!* to be a handbook for enjoyable living. May it inspire you to evaluate your own habits, set new goals for healthier eating, celebrate your victories, and take new steps on the road toward lifelong health.

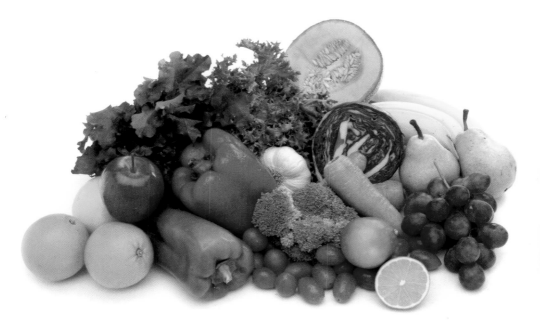

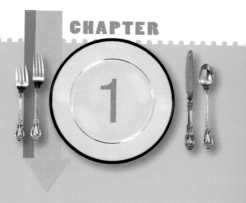

LIVING FOOD VS. DEAD FOOD

Living Food
vs. Dead Food

IN THE INTRODUCTION OF this book I asked you to imagine yourself standing at a crossroads with two arrows pointing in opposite directions: one leading to life and the other leading to death. Does that give you an idea of how serious I think your food choices are? As we begin this chapter, let's try another visual image. Imagine you have two shelves in your pantry, one that says "dead food" and the other "living food."

On the "dead food" shelf is a label that reads: "These foods will increase your risk of developing degenerative diseases such as diabetes, cardiovascular disease, and arthritis, and make you overweight. They will also make you more prone to fatigue, hypertension, and high cholesterol."

But the "living food" shelf's label reads: "These foods will help your body arm itself against cancer, heart disease, degenerative diseases, and obesity, and they will sharpen your mind, energize you, and enliven you."

Which shelf are you going to choose?

Those shelves are not imaginary. They are real. In your pantry, freezer, and fridge right now are foods that lead to life and death. They are probably all mixed together, live foods next to dead

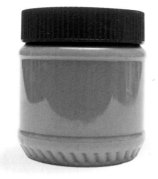

One Timeless Principle of Eating

I'm sure that as more research is done on food and the human body, we will find that some foods may be healthier than we thought (like coffee and dark chocolate). And other foods we considered healthy (such as margarine) are, in fact, harmful to our health.

I once heard a speaker say that after ten years, about half the medical knowledge we have learned turns out to be false. The problem is, we don't know which half!

There will always be changing information regarding foods and their effect on your health, but one timeless principle will always stand: living foods (such as fruits, veggies, and whole grains) will always be healthier for you than processed foods.

foods—processed peanut butter next to extra-virgin olive oil, oatmeal next to an XXL-size bag of potato chips.

As we embark on our journey to understand living foods, you need to realize that everything you put in your mouth has the potential to produce life or death. Food is meant to be savored and enjoyed. But eating the wrong foods will bring poor health and can even shorten your life. Are you at war with your health because of the foods you eat? Or are you enjoying the beautiful dance of hunger and satisfaction that centers around the divine gift of living food?

Living foods will always be healthier than processed foods.

"WHY DOES IT MATTER WHAT I EAT?"

Nutrition Facts

Serving Size 1/2 cup (39g) dry
Servings Per Container about 13

Amount Per Serving	Cereal	Cereal with 1/2 cup Skim Milk
Calories	140	190
Calories from Fat	25	30
	% Daily Value**	
Total Fat 3g*	5%	5%
Saturated Fat 0.5g	3%	3%
Cholesterol 0mg	0%	0%
Sodium 0mg	0%	3%
Total Carbohydrate 26g	9%	11%
Dietary Fiber 4g	16%	16%
Soluble Fiber 2g		
Sugars 0g		
Protein 5g		
Vitamin A	0%	6%
	0%	2%

ALL MEN ARE CREATED equal, but all foods are not! In fact, some food should not be labeled "food" but rather "consumable product" or "edible, but void of nourishment."

Living foods—fruits, vegetables, grains, seeds, and nuts—exist in a raw or close-to-raw state and are beautifully packaged in divinely created wrappers called skins and peels. Living foods look robust, healthy, and alive. They have not been bleached, refined, or chemically enhanced and preserved. Living foods are plucked, harvested, and squeezed—not processed, packaged, and put on a shelf. Living foods are recognizable as food.

Dead foods are the opposite. They have been altered in every imaginable way to make them last as long as possible and be as addictive as possible. That usually means the manufacturer adds considerable amounts of sugar and man-made fats that involve taking various oils and heating them to dangerously high temperatures so that the nutrients die and become reborn as something completely different—a deadly, sludgy substance that is toxic to our bodies.

Life breeds life. Death breeds death. When you eat living foods, the enzymes in their pristine state interact with your digestive enzymes. The other natural ingredients God put in them—vitamins, minerals, phytonutrients, antioxidants, fiber, and more—flow into your system in their natural state. These living foods were created to cause your digestive system, bloodstream, and organs to function at optimum capacity.

Dead foods hit your body like a foreign intruder. Chemicals, including preservatives, food additives, and bleaching agents, place a strain on the liver. Toxic man-made fats begin to form in your cell membranes; they become stored as fat in your body and form plaque in your arteries. Your body does its best to harvest the tiny traces of good from these deadly foods, but in the end you are undernourished, overfed, and overweight.

If you want to be a healthy, vibrant, energetic person rather than someone bouncing between all-you-can-eat buffets and fast-food restaurants, take your diet seriously. Now is the time to make the change to living foods.

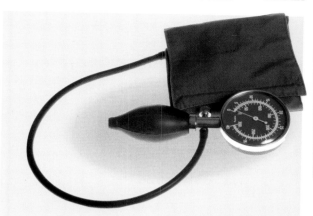

The Twenty-Minute Rule

It takes about twenty minutes for the food you've eaten to reach your small intestines and signal your brain to stop eating. If you stuff yourself with dead foods, it can take even longer for your brain to detect that it has the nutrition it needs. You keep eating more of the same dead foods, and you are caught in a toxic trap.

Living Longer—but Better?

Life expectancy in the United States increased to 77.6 years in 2003, according to a report by the National Center for Health Statistics at the CDC. But half of U.S. residents ages fifty-five to sixty-four have high blood pressure, and two in five are obese.[1]

A Lifetime of Eating

As an average American, you will consume five pounds of food today.[2] Over your lifetime, that's around seventy tons of food that pass through your intestinal tract and are assimilated by your body. This is the equivalent of about forty midsized cars!

YOUR BODY IS A TEMPLE

WONDERFULLY MADE

BEFORE THE FINGER OF God touched the oceans with creative power, God envisioned you in His heart. You are His masterpiece, designed according to an eternal plan so awesome that it's beyond our ability to comprehend. Your body is an amazing creation—something far superior to anything developed by man. Only God Himself could have created such a remarkable work of art. We not only have a body that functions with billions of parts, but we are also blessed with feelings and emotions. The psalmist wrote, "Thank you for making me so wonderfully complex! Your workmanship is marvelous—how well I know it" (Ps. 139:14, NLT).

You were not placed on Earth to be anemic, feeble, and helpless. God wants you to live "more abundantly"—disease free and in maximum health. Your physical body is precious and was created as a dwelling place for your Creator.* Yet most people pollute their temples by eating too much food and eating the wrong foods.

The 2004 movie *Super Size Me* chronicled one man's switch to an all-McDonald's diet. In just thirty days he went from 185 to 209 pounds, his cholesterol went up a whopping 65 points, and his body fat jumped from 11 to 18 percent. That's not even including what

* See 1 Corinthians 3:16; 6:20.

he suffered from mood swings, high blood pressure, and symptoms of addiction. His was an experiment, but many people treat their bodies that way regularly.

If you say, "Everyone around me eats 'bad' food, and they all look fine," consider that maybe everyone around you is unhealthy, in the process of becoming overweight, and disease-prone.

Maybe you have felt hopeless or even said, "Why try now when I've already tried everything?" You said it; *you tried*. The good news is that *you are not alone*. Start practicing temperance, moderation, portion control, and self-restraint when it comes to food. Then, when you make positive changes to your diet, it will have a real and lasting effect on your health.

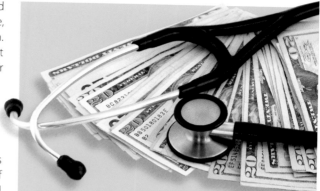

The Hidden Costs of a Value Meal

Many people think that it's cheaper to eat a high-fat, high-calorie fast-food diet than it is to eat healthily. But when you factor in the direct costs (medical costs of obesity have reached $93 billion a year in the United States) and the indirect costs (higher jet fuel costs for airlines transporting heavier passengers, more money spent on gas by the obese themselves), you suddenly realize that supersizing a meal at McDonald's, Burger King, or Kentucky Fried Chicken costs a whole lot more than the extra change you pull out of your pocket.[1]

WHY WE EAT THE WRONG FOODS

THERE ARE MANY CAUSES for unhealthy eating habits. Some are biological, and some are psychological. Over the years, I've heard my patients describe many reasons for their unhealthy food choices. Here are the most common ones:

1. *It's a habit to eat bad foods.* Some people are raised on regional/ethnic cooking that isn't always healthy.

2. *It's convenient to eat bad foods.* To my knowledge, there isn't a health-food drive-through chain or take-out restaurant in America.

3. *It's a vicious cycle.* People fall into a cycle of eating sugar, and the cycle perpetuates itself. When you eat a doughnut, you get a sugar rush, but several hours later your blood-sugar level drops, and you crave a sweet or starchy pick-me-up.

4. *Hormones make bad foods look good.* The fluctuations in hormone levels during pregnancy, PMS, and menopause can cause women to crave sweets and chocolate.

5. *It's comforting to eat bad foods.* Excessive stress elevates cortisol, which leads to cravings and what is often called "emotional eating." When people are stressed, depressed, anxious, or just low in serotonin, norepinephrine, or dopamine, they often reach for foods that pump up these feel-good chemicals. Too often, however, these foods are junk foods, processed foods, and foods high in sugar, making them unhealthy choices.

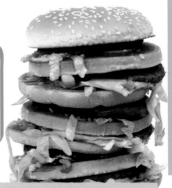

Did You Know...?

People who restrict their calories live longer. More than two thousand studies support the fact that a low-calorie, optimal-nutrition diet can extend life by 30 to 50 percent.[2]

A Nation of Diabetics

A new study indicates that more than one out of three Americans has either impaired fasting glucose (prediabetes) or diabetes. Incidence of diabetes was estimated at 9.3 percent of the population, and impaired fasting glucose at 26 percent of the population. Impaired fasting glucose increases the risk of diabetes.[3]

Comfort Foods Affected by Gender, Age, and Mood

According to Brian Wansink, author of *Mindless Eating*, men and women have different ideas when it comes to comfort foods. The men in Wansink's study were more likely to consider warm meals as comfort foods (pizza, pasta, soup, and steak were among the highest ranked). While women also liked these warm foods, they ranked sweet snack foods (ice cream, candy, chocolate, and cookies) higher on their list of preferences.

Age also played a role. The study found that younger people were more likely to choose potato chips or cookies as comfort foods, and older people were more likely to choose warm meals.

Wansink's research also found that not only do people turn to comfort foods when they are feeling low and need a boost of serotonin, but they also seek out comfort foods when they are happy. The interesting difference is the types of food they choose depending on their mood. According to Wansink, people tend to gravitate toward the healthier options on the comfort foods list when they are celebrating or rewarding themselves (steak or pizza), but when sad, they choose ice cream, cookies, or a bag of potato chips.[4]

Feeling guilty? Don't! Blaming yourself for food cravings can worsen your mood and increase your need for serotonin, setting you up for a pattern of emotional eating.

FOOD CRAVINGS

HAVE YOU EVER CRAVED certain foods and felt that somehow this was a bad reflection on you? Unhealthy food cravings do require an extra measure of self-control if we are going to conquer them, but be encouraged. These cravings are merely your body's way of signaling that something is out of whack. And that "something" can be physical, hormonal, neurochemical, emotional, or even spiritual.

From now on, commit your cravings to God at the moment they occur. He will give you the strength to get through them without overeating and the wisdom to understand what your body or heart is trying to tell you. Let your cravings begin a process of bringing your body back into physical and spiritual balance.

One of the main emotional motivators that can send you running for the fridge is stress. When you hold on to stress and worries, you can become depressed. All of these emotions can lead to overeating as you turn to food for comfort. The sidebar on the next page gives you a few practical tips to help you tame your food cravings while you learn to deal with the underlying emotions that may be causing you to turn to unhealthy foods. On page 14, you will find more information about the mind-body-spirit connection and its effects on your food choices.

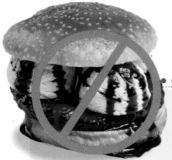

Conquer Your Cravings

Here are a few practical tips to help you curb unhealthy food cravings:

1. Never go anywhere without packing a healthy snack such as fruit or nuts in single-serving-size resealable bags or containers.

2. Keep water with you at all times. Drinking water can often curb hunger pangs and make you feel full without turning to unhealthy foods or high-sugar beverages.

3. Think of a healthier alternative. For instance, instead of a bowl of ice cream, try a scoop of frozen yogurt; instead of potato chips and French onion dip, try baked chips and fresh salsa. While these alternatives might not be ideal, they are a step in the right direction and can help bridge the gap between where you've been and where you want to be with your diet.

4. Control your portions. If you do slip up and indulge in an unhealthy food, never eat directly from the package. Place a small portion on a plate and put the rest away. Challenge yourself to leave part of the food on the plate when you're through, or see if you can move on after only a bite or two.

5. Keep track of your cravings. This can be a key to determining the underlying emotions such as stress that may be causing you to turn to food at certain times of the day, week, or month.

6. Distract yourself. Taking a brisk walk will not only help to get your mind off of your craving, but it will also release stress and burn off some calories in the process. Calling a friend is calorie free and fat free, and a much healthier source of comfort than a tub of Ben & Jerry's.

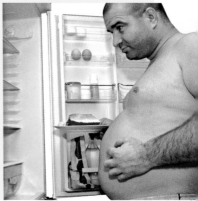

7. Eat three well-balanced meals a day and a healthy midafternoon snack. Consume high-fiber foods with each meal and snack. This will help stabilize blood sugar and help to control hunger.

THE MIND-BODY-SPIRIT CONNECTION

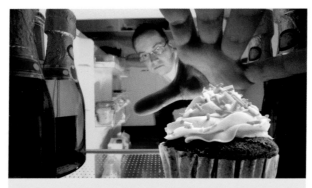

Possible Reasons Behind Emotional Eating

If eating has an emotional component in your life, you probably grew up hearing statements like the following:

- "Eat something; it will make you feel better."

- "Clean your plate or you can't leave the table."

- "If you're good, you'll get dessert."

- "If you don't eat everything on your plate, you are being rude to the person who prepared your meal."

- "If you stop crying, I'll give you some ice cream."

The list of unhealthy childhood motivations for eating is endless. But whether the causes of your eating habits are genetic or psychological, you are not bound by your past. Today is a new day filled with fresh hope for a new way of thinking and living. Start by evaluating what life-style factors might be contributing to your situation.

MANY TIMES PEOPLE WHO struggle with unhealthy eating habits or weight problems experience self-loathing, loneliness, low self-esteem, depression, guilt, and shame, especially the latter two. Over the years, I have treated numerous patients, and I've found that whether their issues with food result in being overweight or underweight, almost always the root cause is emotional. The moment they mess up by eating something they shouldn't, they feel guilty and ashamed, and they feel like quitting.

In my medical office, we know that we need to treat the patient's body, mind (emotions), and spirit. We give them scriptures to confess aloud daily and meditate upon so that they begin to change their mind-set from a negative to a positive state. The Word of God gives them hope.

Often I take these patients through something I call "forgiveness therapy," which enables them to forgive themselves as well as others. When they forgive themselves and begin to love, respect, and accept themselves, it breaks the vicious cycle of negative feelings and emotions. Then and only then do we address the patient's physical needs by making lifestyle changes like eating living foods and exercising.

Perhaps reading this has struck a chord deep within you. For the first time, you may be realizing the connection between some unresolved issues in your past and your current struggle to control your eating habits. You must be willing to start loving yourself and forgiving yourself. In so doing, you can begin to exercise self-control over your physical body and its cravings. I encourage you to read my book *The Seven Pillars of Health* to learn more about the power of forgiveness.

I am praying for God to give you the determination and willpower to follow through on the new eating strategies you are forming as you read this book. Not only will you lose weight and feel better, but you will also be taking care of your body, God's temple, and begin to live a full and abundant life.

Eating Disorders

Eating disorders must not be taken lightly. If your daily life is affected by your struggles with food or body image—whether your weight is impacted or not—I urge you to talk to someone or visit Web sites such as www.nationaleatingdisorders.org for resources that can help you.

A new eating disorder has recently been identified and is on the rise: orthorexia. Orthorexia occurs when someone develops a phobia of eating unhealthy foods. I encourage patients experiencing this disorder to:

- Realize that fear does not come from God (2 Tim. 1:7).

- Remember that moderation is the key. All of the dietary recommendations I make in my books are to be used with moderation and balance. It is never healthy to take these cautions or recommendations to the extreme.

  I also encourage people with fear of unhealthy foods to realize that eating living foods is only one of seven pillars of health. Managing stress (created by fears and worries) is another pillar for healthy living. I go into this in more detail in my books *The Seven Pillars of Health* and *Stress Less*.

  Again, if your thoughts and actions are being affected by an unhealthy fixation on eating, I encourage you to seek professional help.

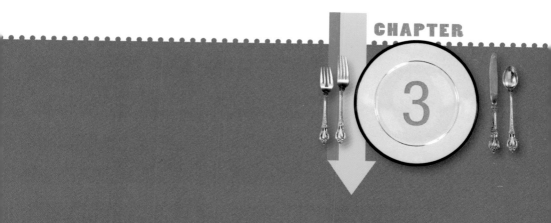

WHAT THE BIBLE SAYS ABOUT FOOD

GOD'S PLAN FOR OUR DIET

PATIENTS OFTEN ASK ME if God wanted humans to be vegetarians. The answer is yes *and* no. Originally, vegetarianism was His design for all people and animals.

> And God said, "See, I have given you every herb that yields seed which is on the face of the earth, and every tree whose fruit yields seed; to you it shall be for food. And to every beast of the earth, to every bird of the air, and to everything that creeps on the earth, in which there is life, I have given every green herb for food"; and it was so.
>
> —GENESIS 1:29–30

That plan changed when the Lord said to Noah, "Every moving thing that lives shall be food for you. I have given you all things, even as the green herbs" (Gen. 9:3). The only exception was this: "But you shall not eat flesh with its life, that is, its blood" (v. 4). That opened up the entire world of living things as a smorgasbord for man's eating pleasure.

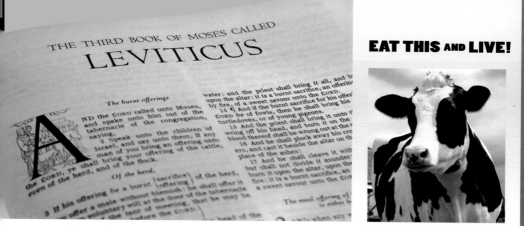

But in Leviticus 11 and Deuteronomy 14, the Lord gave instructions through Moses about how to eat healthily. He said which animals, birds, and fish to eat. For example, they were only allowed to eat animals that chewed cud and had split hoofs, such as cows, sheep, and goats.

The Jews lived under those rules for centuries, and their bodies were strong and disease resistant. The Bible says there was none feeble among all two million Jews in the wilderness (Ps. 105:37). Their phenomenal health plan was based on diet alone!

Jesus also abided by those same rules, never eating pork, shellfish, catfish, or other restricted foods. He was certainly not a vegetarian, but as an observant Jew He would have followed the dietary laws God gave to Moses.

After Jesus's death and resurrection, the dietary rules radically changed, and we are no longer under the law but under grace.

> For everything God created is good, and nothing is to be rejected if it is received with thanksgiving, because it is consecrated by the word of God and prayer.
>
> —1 TIMOTHY 4:4–5, NIV

The apostles and elders also gave their recommendations (Acts 15:28–29) about not eating food that has been sacrificed to idols, or eating blood or the meat of animals that have been strangled. But nowhere did they say to follow the dietary laws of Leviticus 11 or Deuteronomy 14.

As a Christian, you are free to eat anything you want. Your diet will not keep you from heaven, but if you continually eat unhealthy foods, you will get there much sooner. As Paul wrote, all things are permissible, but not all things are beneficial. (See 1 Corinthians 6:12.) We must choose a diet that is good for us. Christians are supposed to be "living epistles." Non-Christians should look at us and visibly see a difference, not only in our attitude but also in our very appearance, which begins with what we eat.

BACK TO BASICS

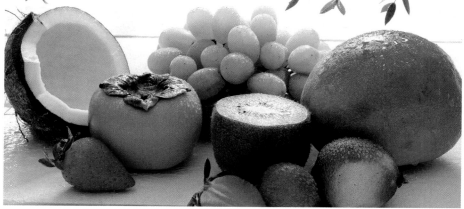

IF GOD IS THE same yesterday, today, and forever, as Hebrews 13:8 says, then what is the wisest diet for us to follow? I believe God's initial plan for vegetarianism, His first and best plan for mankind, should carry a lot of weight with us. I don't promote strict vegetarianism—and neither does God; after all, He told Peter, "Rise, Peter; kill and eat" (Acts 10:13)—but I do note that vegetarians live longer and may have lower incidences of heart disease and cancer.

The Bible itself gives a real-life example of vegetarianism's benefits. In the Book of Daniel, Daniel and three other Jewish youths in the king's palace in Babylon were to be educated and nourished for three years on the king's own rich food and wine. But Daniel would not defile himself by eating the food and wine, because if he did so, he would be breaking the Mosaic laws of Leviticus 11 and Deuteronomy 14. He and his three friends were allowed to shun the king's food and eat pulse (vegetables; grains like wheat, barley, and rye; peas; beans; lentils) for ten days. After ten days, they looked better and

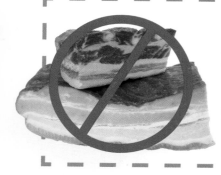

Carnivores, Beware!

A significant study of Seventh-Day Adventists who ate little or no meat showed increased longevity of life of 7.28 years in men and 4.42 years in women.[1]

Another study showed that vegetarians under the age of sixty-five were 45 percent less likely to suffer a heart attack than meat eaters.[2]

healthier than all the other youths. Three years later Daniel and his three friends stood before King Nebuchadnezzar and were ten times wiser than all the magicians and astrologers in the kingdom.

That's a pretty good testimony for eating vegetables, grains, and water.

Please don't misinterpret what I am saying; I am not advocating cutting meat out entirely. When people begin to command you to abstain from certain meats, realize that every creature of God is good, and you can have it as long as you bless it:

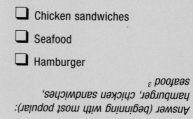

Quick Quiz

Put these top three take-out foods in order of popularity among men in the United States:

☐ Chicken sandwiches

☐ Seafood

☐ Hamburger

Answer (beginning with most popular): hamburger, chicken sandwiches, seafood 3

Now the Spirit expressly says that in latter times some will depart from the faith...commanding to *abstain from foods which God created* to be received with thanksgiving by those who believe and know the truth. For *every creature of God* is good, and nothing is to be refused if it is received with thanksgiving.

—1 TIMOTHY 4:1–4, EMPHASIS ADDED

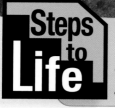

The key here is to practice balance and moderation, especially when eating meats. Also, realize that this scripture refers to foods God created. The foods that are causing disease and killing Americans are foods such as processed foods, fast foods, and foods high in sugar and toxic man-made fats and oils. Eating the right foods makes you physically healthy and wise. Eat the wrong foods, and you open the door to degeneration, disease, and an early death.

Steps to Life

Ask yourself this question: *What would Jesus eat?* Beginning today, get back to the basics.

- Increase your intake of fruits, vegetables, and healthy nuts.
- Choose whole-grain breads over white breads.

WHAT TO AVOID

THE DARK SIDE OF THE FOOD WORLD

I REALIZE THAT FOR the next several pages of this book, I am giving you a lot of information, but it is information that is vitally important for you to understand. If you only come away with one concept from this chapter, I want you to understand that the foods we need to avoid are not necessarily the "unclean foods" listed in Leviticus and Deuteronomy; the foods we need to avoid because they are causing the epidemic of obesity and disease are the man-made foods—processed foods, fast foods, excessive sugars, and toxic fats. These foods are the real killers in the American diet.

Junk-food junkies?

According to a National Health and Nutrition Examination Survey (NHANES), one-third of the average American diet is junk food.[1]

Did You Know…?

According to statistics published by the FAO (the United Nations' Food and Agriculture Organization), the average American eats 3,770 calories per day![2]

Sue's Story

A patient of mine named Sue had been overweight all of her life. Every year as I performed her physical exam, I would recommend weight loss and an exercise program.

At age forty-five, Sue was 5 feet 2 inches, and her weight had climbed to 300 pounds. At her exam that year, after diagnosing her with hypertension, high cholesterol, and type 2 diabetes, I repeated my recommendations for weight loss and exercise.

Sue laughed and said, "My whole family is fat. My dad is fat and he is alive, my mom is fat and she's alive, and my brother and sister are fat and they are alive. Just give me my meds, because I'm sure not going to give up my ice cream each evening, my Krispy Kreme doughnuts every morning, or my burgers, pizza, fried chicken, french fries, and Coke. Besides, I just love to eat."

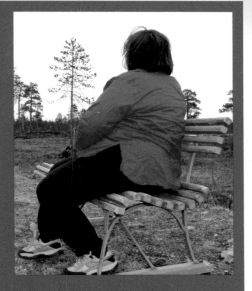

A few months after that physical, Sue suffered a massive heart attack and almost died. She had a quadruple bypass and found herself lying in the hospital with all sorts of tubes coming out of her body. After getting out of the hospital, Sue followed up with me in my office. She said that the pain and possibility of dying and not seeing her three children grow up were not worth the pleasure of eating ice cream, doughnuts, or fast foods.

Nearly dying was a wake-up call for Sue to change her bad habits. She lost 150 pounds—that's half her body weight—in two years and now weighs 150 pounds. She weighs herself every day, and if she gains one or two pounds, she loses them by modifying her diet and activities.

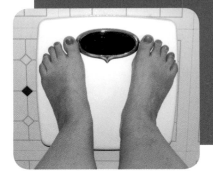

You do not have to wait for a near-death experience like Sue's to serve as your wake-up call; you can start taking your health more seriously right now. The same choice God gave His people centuries ago is yours to make today: "I have set before you life and death, blessing and cursing; therefore choose life, that both you and your descendants may live" (Deut. 30:19).

THE PLAGUE OF PROCESSED FOODS

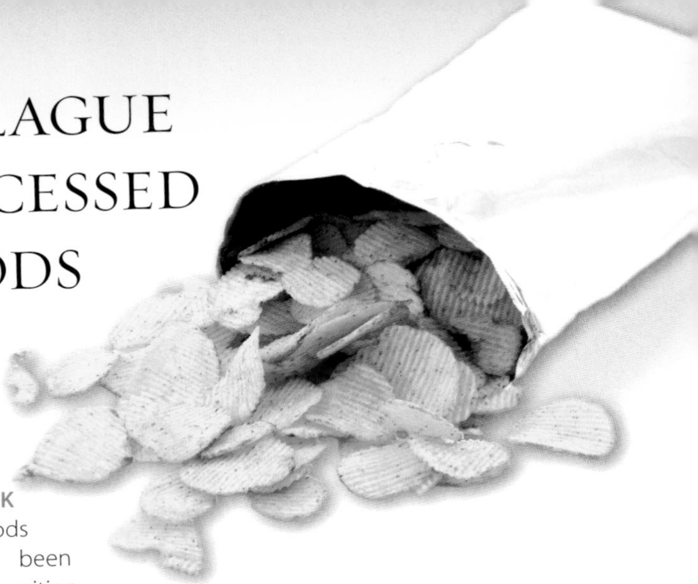

EARLIER IN THIS BOOK I described dead foods as those that have been processed beyond recognition. Dead foods have had the life sucked out of them and man-made chemicals added to extend their shelf life. I like to call them "Franken-foods." Your first rule of thumb is this: limit your intake of dead, processed food (white bread, instant white rice, crackers, chips, and so forth). It enriches the food company's bottom line but usually constipates your body. If processing food made it healthier, I would be its biggest advocate, but processed foods are—without exception—higher in toxic fats, depleted flours, sugar, salt, and food additives.

The man-made process that produces this "Franken-food" strips away valuable vitamins, minerals, fiber, enzymes, phytonutrients, and antioxidants. Most processed foods have a high glycemic index and raise your blood sugar, causing

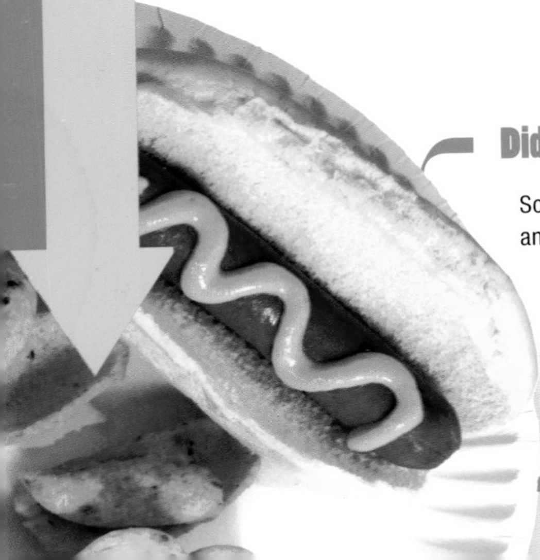

Did You Know...?

Some of the most commonly consumed foods and beverages in America are:

- White bread
- Prepared cereals
- Milk
- Soft drinks[3]

weight gain and setting the stage for most degenerative diseases. Most contain little to no nutrition and actually put a strain on your digestive enzymes.

To make matters worse, food companies make these processed foods as addictive as possible so you'll keep coming back for more. They hire the smartest chemists to create foods that look, taste, feel, sound, and smell irresistible. Then they hire the brightest marketers to package and promote their products in a way that appeals to you and your children—like putting toys in cereal boxes and cartoon characters on the outside of the packages.

But it's time for you to boot dead foods out of your life. On the next several pages I will explain the main processed foods you need to kick out or reduce dramatically.

Processed Foods, Fast Foods, and Poor Health

I am convinced that the following fourteen health conditions are brought on primarily through the intake of large amounts of processed foods.

1. Acid reflux disease
2. Arthritis
3. Addictions
4. Attention deficit disorder
5. Cancer
6. Chronic fatigue syndrome
7. Diabetes
8. Diverticulitis and diverticulosis
9. Fibromyalgia
10. Gallbladder disease
11. Heart disease
12. High cholesterol
13. Hypertension (high blood pressure)
14. Obesity

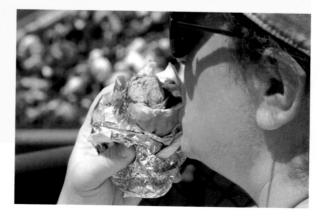

CHEMICAL-LADEN FOODS

From the lab to the lunchroom: Just how many chemicals are in your food?

ALMOST ALL NONORGANICALLY GROWN produce may be tainted by pesticides, herbicides, parasites, and chemicals. These toxins and microbes find their way into our food supply—and into our bodies.

Pesticides are absorbed in the intestinal tract from an animal's feed, and what is not detoxified by the animal's liver may be deposited in their fatty tissues. When you eat meat, it eventually goes into your fatty tissues—including your brain.

If you eat processed foods, you welcome a host of chemicals into your body, including synthetic dyes, flavoring agents, chemical preservatives, emulsifiers, texturizers, humectants, bleaching agents, and sugar substitutes like aspartame. Chemical food additives are usually made from—brace yourself—petroleum or coal tar products. Bleaching agents can be so toxic that Germany has banned their use in flour since 1958.[4]

One of the most toxic bleaching agents used is chloride oxide, also known as chlorine dioxide. When this chemical agent

Pesticides Linked to Disease

Pesticide exposure changes areas of the brain involved in multiple sclerosis, epilepsy, and Alzheimer's disease.[5]

A study of 143,000 people found those exposed to pesticides had a 70 percent higher incidence of Parkinson's disease.[6]

Farmers who have been exposed to pesticides have increased incidence of leukemia, non-Hodgkin's lymphoma, multiple myeloma, soft-tissue sarcoma, and other cancers.[7]

combines with the proteins that are left after the bran and germ are removed from the wheat, it forms a substance called alloxan. Alloxan may trigger selective destruction of beta cells in the pancreas, potentially causing type 2 diabetes.[8] Despite this, the FDA still allows companies to use this bleaching agent in foods.

Some toxic chemicals, such as DDT and PCBs, have been banned in the United States for decades, but since these chemicals remain in our water, land, and air, fish and animal products continue to be main sources of DDT and PCBs in our diets. The EPA lists DDT and PCBs as probable human carcinogens since both cause liver cancer in laboratory animals.[9]

These chemicals are stored in an animal's fat, so the best way to reduce your risk of ingesting chemicals is to choose lean cuts of organic meat and low-fat organic dairy products. Avoid sport-caught fish (such as swordfish) and shellfish, which are often high in DDT and PCBs. Commercial fish that are high in PCBs include Atlantic or farmed salmon, bluefish, wild striped bass, white and Atlantic croaker, blackback or winter flounder, summer flounder, and blue crab. Commercial fish that contain higher levels of pesticides, including DDT, are bluefish, wild striped bass, American eel, and Atlantic salmon. When preparing your meal, broil or bake your fish to allow as much fat as possible to drain from it. See page 102 for a list of fish I recommend eating.

Fighting the FDA on Food Dyes[10]

Thanks to FDA approval of certain food dyes, the amount of dye consumed by American children has increased from 12 mg per day in 1955 to 59 mg per day in 2007. But in June 2008, the Center for Science in the Public Interest petitioned the FDA to ban eight synthetic food dyes, claiming they cause hyperactivity and other behavioral problems in children. The food dyes listed in the petition include Yellow 5 and Red 40, the two most common dyes used in the United States, along with Green 3, Orange B, Blue 1, Red 3, Blue 2, and Yellow 6. Common cereals and candies that contain one or more of these questionable food dyes are:

- Apple Jacks
- Froot Loops
- Fruity Cheerios
- Lucky Charms
- Fruity Pebbles
- Trix
- Starburst Chews
- Skittles
- M&Ms

Did You Know…?

Soft drinks are practically pesticide free. But they contain far too much sugar to have any health benefit, and diet drinks usually contain aspartame, which chemically breaks down to methanol. Also, they are high in phosphates, which are associated with calcium loss.

MSG

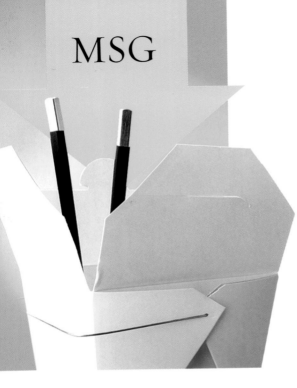

A COMMON INGREDIENT IN processed foods—as well as one of the most dangerous and best disguised—is MSG (monosodium glutamate). MSG is the sodium salt of an amino acid, glutamic acid, and looks similar to sugar or salt. MSG doesn't alter the actual taste of food the way salt and other seasonings do. Instead it "enhances" taste by increasing the sensitivity of your taste buds.

Most of our MSG intake comes from processed foods. Not only is it hidden in most of the store-bought processed foods, but it is also in many of the processed foods in restaurants, such as fried chicken products, sausage, scrambled egg mix, and grilled chicken fillet.

So why the big fuss over MSG? We've known about some of the

Adverse Reactions Caused by MSG

Here is a sampling of some of the reactions that MSG-sensitive people may experience within an hour of ingesting 3 grams of free glutamic acid on an empty stomach:[11]

- Stomach cramps
- Nausea/vomiting
- Diarrhea
- Migraine headaches*
- Heart palpitations
- Rapid heartbeat
- Extreme rise or drop in blood pressure

- Shortness of breath
- Pain or tightness in the chest*
- Facial swelling*
- Numbness/burning in and around the mouth*
- Frequent urination
- Depression

- Anxiety/panic attacks
- Light-headedness/loss of balance/dizziness
- Joint pain/stiffness
- Flu-like achiness
- Blurry vision

Chinese restaurant syndrome is usually diagnosed when, after eating Chinese food, people experience the symptoms above that have been marked with an asterisk (*). MSG has been implicated (but not proven) to be the cause of this condition.[12]

symptoms when consumed in large quantities, but there are new conditions associated with MSG—obesity and excitotoxicity.

Research confirms that MSG consumed by lab animals causes brain lesions of the hypothalamus. Neuroscientists generally agree that glutamic acid (present in MSG) is neurotoxic and kills neurons by exciting them to death. The very young are most susceptible.

MSG damages the hypothalamus, which controls appetite. A damaged hypothalamus can lead to

a runaway appetite. MSG also causes the pancreas to produce more insulin. The blood sugar often drops due to the excessive insulin and typically makes you hungry. That's why many people are hungry an hour or so later after eating food containing MSG.

The FDA now requires that the ingredient "monosodium glutamate" be listed on food labels. However,

labels can be deceiving. Food manufacturers are getting more creative with their labeling of MSG. Now it comes under the guise of names like hydrolyzed vegetable (or plant) protein, autolyzed yeast, yeast extract, soy protein isolate, natural flavors, artificial flavors, and autolyzed plant protein, to name a few. MSG is found in at least thirty-six common label ingredients.

Rule of Thumb

Generally, the more salty or processed a food is, the more MSG or "free glutamate" the food contains.

HIDDEN SOURCES OF MSG

These ingredients ALWAYS contain MSG:

Glutamate	Textured protein	Yeast extract
Glutamic acid	Hydrolyzed protein	Yeast food
Monosodium glutamate	Calcium caseinate	Autolyzed yeast
Monopotassium glutamate	Sodium caseinate	Gelatin

These ingredients OFTEN contain MSG or create MSG during processing:

Articifial flavors and flavorings	Seasonings	Natural flavors and flavorings
Soy sauce	Soy protein isolate	Soy protein
Bouillon	Stock	Broth
Malt extract	Malt flavoring	Barley malt
Whey protein	Carrageenan	Maltodextrin
Pectin	Enzymes	Protease
Corn starch	Citric acid	Powdered milk
Protein-fortified ingredients	Enzyme-modified ingredients	Ultra-pasteurized ingredients

HIGH-SUGAR FOODS AND BEVERAGES

REFINED SUGAR IS A man-made product, unlike the natural sugars found in living food.

Why is sugar so harmful?

1. Sugar is addictive.

Many people find it nearly impossible to stop eating sugar. In fact, eating lots of sugar may deplete the zinc in your body, which can dull your sense of taste.[13] When your taste perception is altered, you need more sugar to give you the same taste satisfaction. It becomes a vicious cycle.

2. Sugar can impair your immune system.

Eating 100 grams of simple carbohydrates (like cookies, a large piece of cake, or a few doughnuts) can reduce the ability of white blood cells by 50 percent for a few hours.

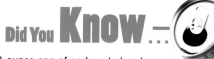

Did You Know...

A 12-ounce can of carbonated soda contains 8–10 teaspoons of sugar.[14]

3. Sugar is linked to behavioral disorders.

There's a strong link between excessive sugar intake and attention-deficit hyperactivity disorder (ADHD). Some authorities have even linked sugar and hypoglycemia (low blood sugar) with violent behavior.[15] They believe that when individuals "come down" from a sugar "high," they become grumpy, irritable, and may even become violent.

EAT THIS AND LIVE!

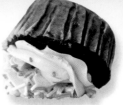

4. Sugar can lead to osteoporosis.

Sugar creates an acidic environment in your tissues, which causes your body to cry out for alkaline foods. If you don't get enough calcium in your diet, your body may pull it from your bones and teeth to rebalance your pH, and you may develop bone loss and eventually osteoporosis.

5. Sugar can lead to type 2 diabetes and elevate cholesterol.

Most people understand how sugar excess can lead to diabetes by elevating insulin levels; eventually cells become resistant to insulin, which leads to type 2 diabetes. But elevated insulin levels also trigger the liver to produce more cholesterol and triglycerides.

Sugar Overload

Back in the 1980s the average American ate 6 tablespoons of sugar a day. Ten years later, that average was 16 tablespoons of sugar. As of 2005, the average American consumes 150 pounds of sugar every year![16]

One reason is that "stealth sugar" is added to many products. Check the basic items in your pantry and you will see that sugar is high on the ingredient list. You may be avoiding candy bars but getting just as much sugar in unexpected places. For example, 1 tablespoon of ketchup contains approximately 1 teaspoon of sugar.

6. Sugar can make you fat.

When you overeat sugar, your body goes into fat-storage mode. That's why most diabetics gain weight when they begin taking insulin—often as much as twenty or thirty pounds. Sugar creates a cycle of demand for more sugar, which raises insulin levels. Insulin is a powerful hormone that signals the body to store fat.

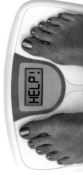

Artificial Sweeteners

DON'T BE FOOLED BY packaging that says "sugar free" or "diet," since this means that somewhere along the way, an artificial sweetener was likely added to the ingredients to make up for the sugar that was removed. The list of health risks associated with consumption of artificial sweeteners is just as alarming as that of sugar. Here's a quick primer on sweeteners.

Aspartame exposed

Aspartame is made of three components: aspartic acid, phenylalanine, and methanol. Methanol is also known as "wood alcohol," and it is 10 percent of what is released from aspartame when this substance is broken down in the human digestive tract. When a beverage containing aspartame is exposed to heat, it releases methanol.

In the body, methanol is converted to formaldehyde—yes, embalming fluid—and formic acid. Methanol and formaldehyde in high amounts can cause blindness, eye damage, or neurological damage.

Side effects of aspartame include vision problems, headaches, confusion, depression, dizziness, convulsions, nausea, diarrhea, migraines, abdominal pain, fatigue, chest tightness, and shortness of breath.

Is Splenda OK?

Splenda brand sweetener is a substance called sucralose, which is made by turning sugar into a chlorocarbon. A few of the side effects of sucralose in animal studies include shrunken thymus glands (the thymus is critical in warding off cancer and infections[17]), enlarged liver and kidneys, atrophy of the lymph follicles in the spleen and thymus, reduced growth rate, decrease in red blood cell count, hyperplasia of the pelvis, aborted pregnancy, decreased fetal body weights and placental weights, and diarrhea.[18]

Some people have reported the conditions listed in the sidebar on the facing page after consuming Splenda. No long-term studies of sucralose in humans have been completed, but according to a laboratory in Oxford, England, sucralose may form trace amounts of a mutagenic agent that may act as a carcinogen.[19]

Remember, I always recommend natural products in place of artificial sweeteners.

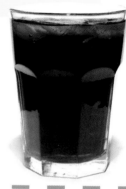

Natural Sweeteners

I recommend that you switch to natural sweeteners like stevia, chicory root, Lo Han, or xylitol. Be careful with xylitol, though, because it may cause excessive gas.

Aspartame in the News...

According to a press release distributed by *Newswire Today* on January 17, 2006, a bill to ban the artificial sweetener aspartame was introduced in the New Mexico legislature by New Mexico state senator Jerry Ortiz y Pino. It is the first legislative ban in the United States on aspartame.

According to the press release, a report posted on the National Institutes of Health Web site in November 2005 stated: "The Ramazzini Foundation of Oncology's study proves aspartame to cause 6 kinds of cancer."[20]

The "Not-So-Splendid" Side of Splenda

People who use Splenda (sucralose) may experience the following side effects:

- Bloating
- Abdominal pain
- Gas
- Nausea
- Blurry vision
- Diarrhea
- Headaches, especially migraines
- Heart palpitations
- Shortness of breath
- Frequent need to urinate at night
- Depression or overwhelming anxiety
- "Spaced-out" or drugged sensation
- Joint pain
- Dizziness[21]

To Diet or Not to Diet Soda?

Many people think diet sodas help them lose weight, but one study showed otherwise. A study covering eight years of collected data showed that your risk of becoming overweight by drinking one to two cans of soda per day is 32.8 percent, but your risk increases to 54.5 percent if you drink one to two cans of diet soda instead.[22]

WHITE FLOUR

MORE THAN LIKELY YOU were given a sandwich made with white bread on a daily basis when you were a kid, but white bread and other products made from refined flour are poor choices for food. Refined white flour is just another example of how a wonderful, God-given food gets mugged on the way to the grocery shelf.

White bread delivers little nutrition (even with all those added vitamins and minerals they advertise on the packages of "enriched" products) and converts to sugar rapidly—almost as fast as a candy bar. When my diabetic patients switch from eating white bread to whole-grain bread, their cholesterol and blood sugars almost always go down.

You can be sure that any flour not labeled as "whole wheat" or "whole grain" is refined white flour, even if it looks brown. That's right, some manufacturers add molasses to the ingredients to give the bread a darker appearance and mislead health-conscious consumers into thinking they are buying whole-grain bread!

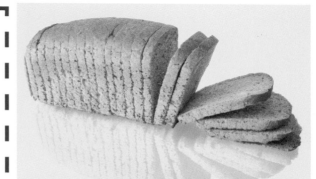

Label Decoder: Whole Grains

It seems that the more we learn about healthy eating, the more food marketers try to con us into thinking their products are good for us. Here's a tip to help you decide whether a bread, cracker, or cereal product is truly whole grain or just an imposter:

As a general rule of thumb, don't trust the words "whole grain" on the front of the package. Instead, read the ingredients. You're probably looking at a whole-grain product if the words "whole wheat," "oats," or "rye" are near the top of the ingredients list.

Words and phrases like "made with whole grain," "multigrain," "oat bran," "stoned wheat," and "unbleached wheat flour" sound healthy, but might be giveaways that you are reading the label of a product made from refined grains. Also, choose a whole-grain bread that has at least 3 grams of fiber per slice. See page 56 for more information on whole grains.

The Journey From Wheat to White

All bread starts out as whole grain, but to make white bread, the manufacturer removes the outer shell of the grain with all its healthy fiber and B vitamins. Then the nutrition-packed wheat germ is extracted. Both the fiber and the wheat germ are actually *resold to health food stores*. Meanwhile, the denuded white flour heads to the mainstream market to be made into white bread, buns, pastries, crackers, pasta, and so on.

White bread is created from one part of the grain head—the starchy endosperm that is ground into fine powder. Since the bran and germ are removed, approximately 80 percent of the wheat's nutrients are gone. The milling process involves such high temperatures that the remaining grain is damaged by oxidation and has a grayish appearance. Could you imagine buying gray-colored bread?

But because consumers don't want to buy gray bread, the manufacturer bleaches it white. If there were any vitamins and minerals left, most are destroyed in the bleaching process. Then low-grade vitamins and minerals are added, along with man-made cyber-fats, sugars, food additives, and maybe a sprinkling of grains on the top, and the food is marketed to moms as healthy sandwich bread.

Fast Food

THE TYPICAL AMERICAN NOW consumes three hamburgers and four orders of fries per week. In 1970 Americans spent approximately $6 billion on fast food, and in 2000, we spent more than $110 billion.[24] We spend more money on fast food than we do on personal computers, computer software, new cars, and higher education combined.

Unhealthy fats are found in especially high amounts in fast food. In February 2006, a report showed that McDonald's french fries were one-third higher in trans fat than once believed. Although they've recently taken steps to remove deadly trans fats from their cooking processes, a medium serving of fries still contains 19 total grams of fat.

Acrylamides are toxic chemicals formed by the combustion of oil and hydrocarbons. They are highly carcinogenic—particularly associated with colon cancer—and should be avoided. Acrylamides cause cellular DNA to mutate. French fries are among the worst offenders when it comes to foods containing acrylamides. So, the next time you're tempted to go to the drive-through, keep on driving!

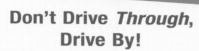

Don't Drive *Through*, Drive By!

Millions of people regularly eat at popular fast-food restaurants. Although many of these restaurants have made great strides in adding healthier fare to their menus in recent years, let's pause for a moment and see what you're really eating when you order something from the list of familiar favorites.

- One thigh of Original Recipe Kentucky Fried Chicken, 20 grams of fat. Make it Extra Crispy and you bump up the fat content to 27 grams. And who doesn't add the mashed potatoes, gravy, and biscuit? Now, you're taking in a total of 660 calories and 40 grams of fat in a single serving.

- If you order a Grilled Stuft Burrito with beef at Taco Bell, you're thinking outside the bun with 680 calories and 30 grams of fat. Switch to chicken and you're not that much better off at 640 calories and 23 grams of fat. (Though chicken is less fatty than beef, this menu item contains saturated and trans fats.)

- Have a Big Mac at McDonald's and you'll rack up 540 calories and 29 grams of fat. The medium french fries contain 380 calories and 19 grams of fat. Even if you decide to be good and drink water, you're still throwing back 920 calories and 48 fat grams.

- Burger King's Whopper contains 670 calories and 39 grams of fat. With cheese added, the fat total rises to 47 grams. Now, make it a combo, and the medium fries add 20 more fat grams. If you include a medium Coke, your total intake for this single meal is 1,330 calories, along with 67 grams of fat.

- A Wendy's Baconator weighs in at 830 calories and 51 grams of fat. Add a medium order of fries and a medium chocolate Frosty and you're eating 1,670 calories and 81 grams of fat in one sitting!

DEADLY (PROCESSED) MEATS

I TRAINED IN A medical residency program operated by Seventh-Day Adventists. As a group they obey certain dietary laws, and many are vegetarians. They also live longer than most Americans and have some of the lowest incidences of heart disease and cancer.[25] Many of them are total vegetarians, eating no meat, fish, fowl, eggs, or dairy products. Some are lacto-ovo vegetarians—meaning they sometimes eat eggs, drink milk, and use other dairy products.

I don't promote total vegetarianism since Jesus was not a vegetarian, but I do believe it's best to limit your intake of certain meats.

- *Livers and kidneys* are filtering organs that filter toxins. Many toxins reside in these organs. Why would you want to eat them?

- *Cold cuts and packaged meats like bologna, salami, and processed ham* are usually high in saturated fats, which are associated with high cholesterol and heart disease and are always high in salt. They also contain lots of nitrites and nitrates— substances that may form cancer-causing chemicals called *nitrosamines* or *n-nitroso compounds*. These compounds are associated with cancer of the bladder, esophagus, stomach, brain, and oral cavity.

  Nitrosamines are formed during digestion when food protein reacts with nitrite salts in the stomach. They can also be formed by frying or smoking. A general rule of thumb is that the more processed and preservative-rich the meat is, the greater the risk of nitrosamines. To lessen this risk, I recommend that you bake your own ham and turkey and slice it yourself instead of picking up cold cuts at the deli.

- *Bacon, sausage, and hot dogs* are also high in saturated fats and chemicals. These meats are generally loaded with saturated fat.

Hot Dog!

It's especially important not to let children eat hot dogs and other processed meats. One study found that children who eat more than twelve hot dogs per month have nine times the normal risk of developing childhood leukemia. Another study found that children who eat hot dogs one or more times per week have a higher risk of developing brain cancer and that children whose mothers ate hot dogs during pregnancy are associated with an excess risk of childhood brain tumors. If hot dogs are a favorite in your household, please switch to brands that say "nitrite-free" or "nitrate-free" on the label.[26] Also, there is nitrite-free bacon, ham, sausage, and luncheon meat.

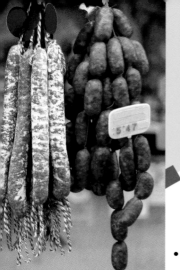

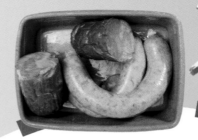

Are Hot Dogs and Sausage Safe?

Whether you call them hot dogs, frankfurters, wieners, or brat-wursts, they're all varieties of cooked sausage, and a few key words on the packaging are your clues to what's really inside:

- Watch for warnings such as "with by-products" or "with variety meats." The USDA requires this wording if the product contains raw meat by-products (e.g., heart, kidney, stomach, intestines, or liver).

- If the product has a casing, watch for artificial colors in the casing. The USDA requires the label to indicate this as well.

- Mechanically separated meat is produced by forcing bones with attached meat through a sieve to separate the bone from the tissue. Mechanically separated *beef* is now prohibited for use as human food due to its connection to mad cow disease, but mechanically separated *pork* and *poultry* are still allowed. Products that exceed the USDA calcium (from bone) content limit must be labeled as containing "mechanically separated" meat.

- Products labeled as "beef franks" or "pork franks" contain meat from a single species and do not contain any animal by-products. However, "turkey franks" or "chicken franks" can contain turkey or chicken meat, turkey or chicken skin and fat, and may contain by-products.[27]

Studies have shown a high level of the harmful bacterial *Listeria* in hot dogs. People at risk (pregnant or nursing women, the elderly, those suffering from a weakened immune system, cancer, diabetes, kidney disease, or AIDS, and those taking certain medications) should avoid eating hot dogs and luncheon meats like bologna.[28]

KILLER TRANS FATS

FATS ADD DELICIOUS TASTE and "mouth feel" to foods, but often at a dangerous price. There are three categories of fats:

1. "Good" fats are living foods (omega-3 fats and monounsaturated fats), and I'll talk about these fats in the next chapter.

2. "OK" fats can kill in excess but heal in moderation (saturated and polyunsaturated fats). Therefore, you need to limit your intake of these fats. Saturated fat is found mostly in animal fats and significantly raises LDL (bad) cholesterol. Polyunsaturated fats are found in products such as mayonnaise, salad dressing, sunflower oil, and corn oil. I'll talk more about these fats on pages 44–45.

3. "Bad" fats are dead foods—they are fats that kill (trans or hydrogenated fats and partially hydrogenated fats). On the facing page, I will explain a little bit about this category of killer trans fats.

I'll talk more about these fats on pages 44–45.

Quick Quiz

Which Bob Evans' menu items contain the highest grams of trans fats?

a. No-sugar-added Apple Pie

b. Turkey and Dressing Dinner

c. Slow-Roasted Chicken Pot Pie

Answer: a and c. The No-sugar-added Apple Pie contains 13 grams of trans fats. The Slow-Roasted Chicken Pot Pie contains 13 grams of trans fats. The Turkey and Dressing contains only 3 grams of trans fats.[29]

During the hydrogenation process, the cheapest oils—soy, corn, cottonseed, and canola—are mixed with a metal catalyst, usually nickel. The oil is then subjected to hydrogen gas in a high-pressure, high-temperature reactor to force hydrogen through it until it is saturated. Emulsifiers are then added, and the oil is deodorized at high temperatures and steam cleaned. Margarine is an example of a product containing hydrogenated oils. Like the white flour I mentioned earlier, margarine must be bleached to hide its gray color and then dyed and flavored to resemble butter.

Adding hydrogen atoms to liquid fats and oils makes these oils stay in solid form at room temperature. This means that they are much less likely to become rancid, and their shelf life is greatly prolonged.

This process, however,

Misleading Labels

On January 1, 2006, all packaged foods sold in the United States began to list trans fat content on their nutrition labels. But under FDA regulations, "if the serving contains less than 0.5 gram [of trans fat], the content, when declared, shall be expressed as zero."[30] That means you could eat several cookies, each with 0.4 grams of trans fats, and end up eating several grams of trans fats even though the label says zero. A fourteen-year study found that just a 2 percent increase in trans fats elevated a person's risk of heart disease by 36 percent.[31] This is such a deadly fat that we need to avoid it entirely. The best way to avoid this is to look for the words "partially hydrogenated" or "shortening" on the label. If either of these words is on the label, don't eat the product.

alters the chemical structure of the fat to an unnatural "trans fatty acid," which becomes an enemy of the heart by raising LDL (bad) cholesterol levels and lowering HDL (good) cholesterol levels. Trans fats have been implicated in heart disease and cancer.

Trans fats are present in margarine, shortening, and most commercial peanut butters. They are found in almost every item in the middle of a grocery store—where all the shelf-stable pastries, rolls, breakfast cereals, breakfast bars, crackers, and processed or packaged foods reside. Bad fats are also found in the bakery section in the doughnuts, pastries, cookies, cakes, pies, and other items that entice you as you walk around the grocery store. Try to avoid the middle aisles and bakeries of the grocery store so that you won't be tempted. Many salad dressings contain hydrogenated fats.

It's a Fact!

The more solid the hydrogenated fat, the more dangerous it is to your body!

SATURATED FATS

SATURATED FATS RARELY CAN be found in fruits and vegetables; they are primarily found in animal products. Foods high in saturated fats include most selections found at fast-food restaurants (hamburgers, chicken strips, and so on), whole-milk products, as well as commercial fried foods and processed foods (cookies, cakes, doughnuts, pies, and pastries).

Saturated fats are also found in cured meat such as bacon, sausage, ham, hot dogs, cold cuts, bologna, salami, and pepperoni. Red meats, duck, and goose meat are also usually quite high in saturated fats. Some vegetable oils such as coconut oil, palm kernel oil, and palm oil are also high in saturated fats.

I recommend limited intake of these fats rather than completely avoiding them because they do provide benefits to the body when consumed in moderation. Saturated

Polyunsaturated Fats: Needed in Small Amounts

Polyunsaturated fats are essential for life and must be consumed. I believe the best way is to consume small portions of pecans, almonds, brazil nuts, pine nuts, pistachios, and walnuts. If you must use vegetable oil, choose small amounts of *cold-pressed* polyunsaturated fats (corn oil, flaxseed oil, hemp oil, pumpkinseed oil, safflower oil, sesame oil, soybean oil, sunflower oil), which you can find at most health food stores. But it's best to avoid *heat-processed* oils and replace your salad dressings with extra-virgin olive oil, balsamic vinegar, and garlic oil, pressed with a garlic press.

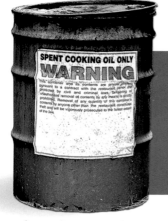

Dr. Colbert's List of Worst Fats to Consume

1. Hydrogenated and partially hydrogenated fats and trans fats

2. Excessive saturated fats

3. Excessive polyunsaturated fats

fats enhance our immune system and allow calcium to be incorporated into our bones when consumed in moderation. *(In moderation means that no more than 7–10 percent of our caloric intake should come from saturated fats.[32])* Moderate amounts of saturated fats also protect the liver from toxins, help prevent breast cancer and colon cancer, and help promote weight loss. Moderation cannot be overstated when talking about saturated fats; for instance, coconut oil is beneficial for weight loss only when you limit it to 1 tablespoon a day (or 1 teaspoon three times a day).

Polyunsaturated fats

Polyunsaturated fats are divided into two families: omega-3 fats and omega-6 fats. I'll discuss omega-3 fats in the next chapter.

When polyunsaturated oils such as corn oil, safflower oil, sunflower oil, sesame oil, commercial salad dressings, and others are used in cooking, and especially deep-frying, oxidation occurs even faster. Oxidation also occurs in your arteries as free radicals attack the polyunsaturated fats, which are carried in LDL cholesterol.

Oxidized cholesterol is much more likely to form plaque in the arteries. As fats are broken down through oxidation, they form substances that promote blood clotting and cause inflammation, making blood flow more difficult.

Polyunsaturated fats are not the worst fats, but they aren't the best, either. They come from healthy sources, but they tend to be overprocessed by the time they reach the consumer. Eating too much polyunsaturated fat increases inflammation, which is associated with heart disease, arthritis, cancer, and Alzheimer's disease.

Did You Know…?

Meat drippings, such as beef tallow/dripping, lard (pork), chicken, duck, goose, bacon fat, and even turkey, contain a whopping 44.8 grams of saturated fat per 3.5 oz serving? So the next time you cook those green beans, think twice about slathering them with bacon fat![33]

STAYIN' ALIVE WITH LIVING FOODS

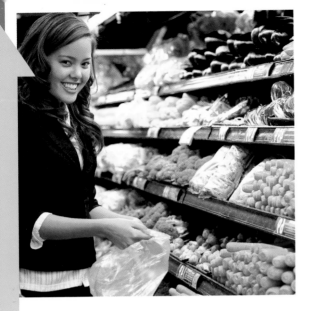

THE LIVING FOODS LIST

IN THE TELEVISION PROGRAM *What Not to Wear*, a crew of hip makeover artists helps a poorly dressed person learn how to dress well. The show ends with the friends and family seeing the transformed person. The before and after photos are often shockingly different.

You "wear" your food on your body every day. You really are what you eat. Your clothes may be made of cotton, polyester, rayon, or silk, but your body is made up of whatever you put in your mouth. Eyeliner and shapers can't hide an unhealthy body. It's time to make over your pantry and fridge with living foods, if only so you can look your best!

Most of us eat what has been called the "standard American diet"—lots of fat, sugar, unhealthy fats, and highly refined wheat products. But we didn't always eat this way. Former generations were some of the

Healing Foods

Hippocrates, the father of medicine, said, "Our food should be our medicine, and our medicine should be our food." In other words, what we eat should be so good for us that it actually heals and restores our bodies. What a difference from the average American mind-set about eating!

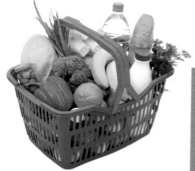

Beauty Is Skin Deep

Organic foods are often smaller and not as pretty as non-organic produce. Organic oranges appear less impressive than conventionally grown ones, but studies show that organic oranges are far more nutrient dense. Nonorganic oranges are bigger and have a nicer orange color, but they are like big balls of water with fewer nutrients.[1]

healthiest on the planet. As an agrarian culture, many of our grandparents lived much closer to the land. But today our lifestyle is much too stressed and fast-paced, and as a result, our diet suffers.

To live healthier, longer lives, we must rethink what we have been taught about food. Food is meant to be enjoyed, but when our dietary choices, which were designed to nourish and sustain our bodies, actually begin to make us ill, then we must change the way we think. On the next several pages you will discover the world of healthy, living foods that bring healing and balance to your body.

In a Nutshell...

Fruits, vegetables, whole grains, and healthy oils are all living food. Not all fats are bad. In fact, your body needs good fat. Good alternatives are extra-virgin olive oil, almonds, macadamia nuts, and flaxseeds. Depending on the oil, you can lightly stir-fry your food, but never deep-fry. I'll discuss these living food options in more detail on the following pages.

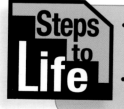

Steps to Life

- Stay on the lighter side of life by enjoying living foods. The more processed and the more sugar and toxic fats a food contains, the more harm it will do to your body.

- Begin reading labels, and choose products with as many whole-food ingredients as possible.

Organic, Free-Range, and Wild-Caught Foods

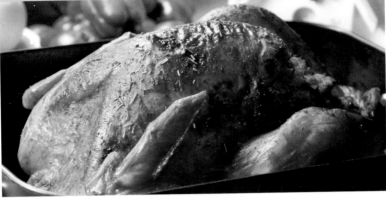

IN ADDITION TO BEING some of the healthiest foods on the planet, produce and live-stock that are developed through organic methods are more eco-friendly, reducing the number of toxins in our land, air, and water. For this reason, a number of people are switching over to organic products in order to live a "greener" life-style. I believe we should be good stewards of our planet; therefore, this is just another great reason for me to recommend organic foods. On these pages, I'll discuss organic produce, free-range meats, and wild-caught seafood.

Exactly What Is "Organic"?

Organic food is defined as having been produced without the use of artificial pesticides and chemical fertil-izers. Not everything that claims to be organically grown is truly organic. Look for this seal, which indicates that the produce has met the USDA's standards for being certi-fied as organically grown.

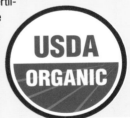

Wild-Caught Fish

One wide-ranging study of farmed salmon vs. wild salmon recom-mended that people eat farmed salmon no more than once a month because of the high toxin content.[2] On average, farmed salmon have 16 times the dioxin-like PCBs found in wild salmon, 4 times the levels in beef, and 3.4 times the dioxin-like PCBs found in other seafood.[3] I recommend avoiding farmed fish altogether; stay on the "wild side" with wild Pacific or Alaskan salmon.

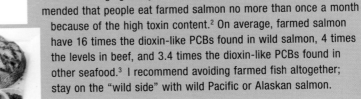

When Organic Produce Is Not Available

Organic produce may not be available in your area, or the selection may be limited or expensive. When nonorganic options are all you have, here are a few rules to remember:

- **Look for thicker peels.** Generally, the thicker the peel or rind, the safer the fruit. For example, bananas have a thick peel; therefore, it is less likely that pesticides are absorbed deeply enough to reach the fruit inside. Oranges, tangerines, lemons, grapefruit, pineapples, watermelons, and figs also have thick peels. You can feel pretty safe purchasing nonorganic selections of these fruits because you remove the peel—and the toxins—before eating.

- **Watch thin peels.** The following thin-peeled produce have been known to carry higher levels of pesticide residue: apples, bell peppers, celery, cherries, imported grapes, nectarines, peaches, pears, potatoes, red raspberries, spinach, and strawberries.[4] Since it is difficult to peel this produce, I strongly recommend organic.

- **Be careful if there's no peel.** What about produce that has no peel, such as lettuce and broccoli? Enjoy your salad, but peel off the outer layer of lettuce leaves if you do not purchase organic. Broccoli can contain higher levels of pesticides, so if you eat a lot of broccoli, purchase an organically grown variety or wash it well.

- **Wash your produce.** You can wash wax off of produce with a natural, biodegradable cleanser or a mild detergent such as pure castile soap.

- **Soak your produce.** Another good way to remove wax and pesticides is to soak produce in a sink of cold water to which you have added 1 tablespoon of 35 percent, food-grade hydrogen peroxide (or 1 teaspoon of Clorox bleach) for five to fifteen minutes. Then rinse thoroughly with fresh water.

Eat Lean Free-Range Meats

Limit your intake of meat and dairy products that have been chemically exposed. Because an animal's body will store pesticides and other chemicals in its fatty tissues, the riskiest foods are fatty cuts of meat. Switch to a leaner cut of meat, and eat free-range or organic meats from cattle grazed on lands that have not been sprayed with pesticides. Free-range organic chicken and turkey are also, for the most part, pesticide- and hormone-free.

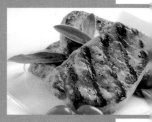

USDA AND OTHER RECOMMENDATIONS

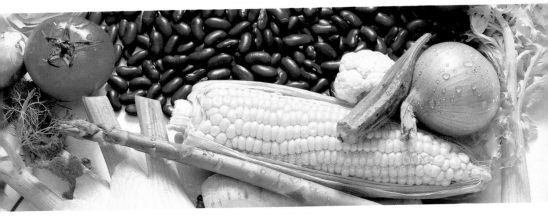

THE U.S. DEPARTMENT OF Agriculture (USDA) has been making dietary recommendations for more than one hundred years. Over time, these recommendations have been adapted to keep up with research findings and changing cultural eating habits. The *Dietary Guidelines for Americans* has been published every five years since 1980 as a collaborative effort between the Department of Health and Human Services (HHS) and the Department of Agriculture (USDA). The 2005 edition of the guidelines included updated recommendations for eating fresh foods. It used to recommend five to seven servings of fruits and vegetables every day. Now it recommends five to thirteen servings a day—almost double the previous recommendations.[5]

The Surgeon General and the National Cancer Institute, along with the USDA and U.S. Department of Health and Human Services, all recommend that we eat plenty of fruits and vegetables. While some studies show that Americans are beginning to consume more vegetables, white potatoes account for 30 percent of the vegetables consumed by Americans, and one-third of these potatoes are french fries.[6] When I recommend you add more vegetables to your diet, believe me, I do not want you to add more french fries!

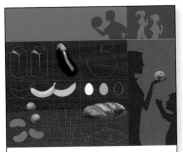

Dietary Guidelines
for Americans
2005

U.S. Department of Health and Human Services
U.S. Department of Agriculture
www.healthierus.gov/dietaryguidelines

Specific vitamins and minerals had not even been discovered yet when the U.S. Department of Agriculture first published a set of dietary recommendations in 1894. Since then, researchers have identified numerous essential vitamins and minerals and established the minimum levels of these nutrients our bodies require in order to prevent deficiencies that can lead to conditions such as scurvy and beriberi.[7]

How Much Is a Serving?

To make sure you eat enough fresh fruits and vegetables each day, it's important to know how much is considered a serving. This can be tricky since the natural "package" your produce comes in doesn't really tell you how much you're eating. The following list shows you how much fresh produce to eat for a ½-cup or a 1-cup serving:

½ Cup Servings	1 Cup Servings
6 cherry tomatoes	12 cherry tomatoes
1 small vine-ripe tomato	2 small vine-ripe tomatoes
½ small cucumber	1 small cucumber
½ large banana	1 large banana
1 slice of cantaloupe (⅛ medium melon)	1 wedge of cantaloupe (¼ medium melon)
6 baby carrots	12 baby carrots
½ medium-size grapefruit or orange	1 medium-size grapefruit or orange
½ bell pepper	1 bell pepper
½ medium apple	1 medium apple
1 plum	2 plums
4 large strawberries	8 large strawberries
1 small potato or sweet potato	1 medium to large potato or sweet potato
5 broccoli spears or cauliflower florets	10 broccoli spears or cauliflower florets
8 grapes	16 grapes
1 small ear of corn	1 large ear of corn

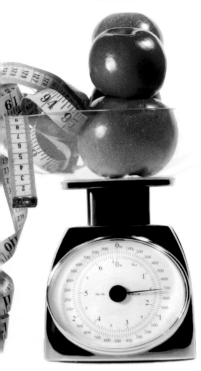

THE GLYCEMIC INDEX

REMEMBER, IN 2005, THE USDA updated its recommendations for eating fresh foods. It used to recommend five to seven servings of fruits and vegetables every day. Now it recommends five to thirteen servings a day—almost double the previous recommendation.

It's hard to go wrong with fresh, organic fruits and vegetables. They should be the major part of your diet. One note of caution, however: fruits and vegetables can be low glycemic or high glycemic. The glycemic index (GI) is a numerical system of measuring how fast a carbohydrate triggers a rise in your blood sugar. The higher the number, the greater the blood sugar response. A low-glycemic food will cause a small rise, while a high-glycemic food will trigger a dramatic spike.

- Low-glycemic foods are 55 or less.
- Medium-glycemic foods are 56–69.
- High-glycemic foods are 70 and above.

I recommend eating produce with a glycemic index of 50 or less. For people trying to lose weight, the chart on the facing page will give you glycemic values for some fruits and vegetables:[8]

Glycemic Index Value	Food
< 15	Artichoke
< 15	Asparagus
< 15	Avocado
< 15	Broccoli
< 15	Cauliflower
< 15	Celery
< 15	Cucumber
< 15	Eggplant
< 15	Green beans
< 15	Lettuce, all varieties
< 15	Peppers, all varieties
< 15	Snow peas
< 15	Spinach
< 15	Young summer squash
< 15	Zucchini
15	Tomatoes
22	Cherries
22	Peas, dried
24	Plum
25	Grapefruit
28	Peach
31	Dried apricots
32	Baby lima beans, frozen
36	Apple
36	Pear
52	Orange juice, not from concentrate
53	Banana
54	Sweet potato
55	Sweet corn
64	Beets
64	Raisins
66	Pineapple
72	Watermelon
97	Parsnips
103	Dates

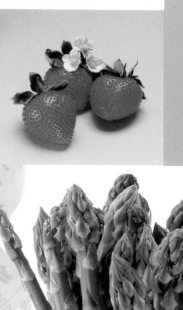

WHOLE GRAINS

ANOTHER LIVING FOODS STAPLE is fiber-rich, living grain products like sprouted-grain breads, brown rice, whole-grain pastas, and whole-grain cereal. Whole-grain products are nutrient-dense and pass on lots of vitamins and minerals to your body. Whole grains also contain lots of fiber, which is a fabulous toxin trapper.

There's no USDA seal of approval for whole grains as there is for organic food. However, an organization called the Whole Grains Council created an official packaging stamp in 2005. The Whole Grain Stamp helps you to know how much whole-grain content various products contain.

There are two versions of the stamp, each clearly noting the product's whole-grain content in grams per serving. The 100% Whole Grain Stamp indicates that all of the grain in a product is whole grain and that you'll enjoy a full serving (16 grams) or more of whole grain when you consume the serving size printed on the label. The Basic Whole Grain Stamp is for products that may also contain some refined grain, but that guarantee you at least half a serving of whole grain per labeled serving.

The Whole Grain Stamp doesn't yet appear on all whole-grain foods, so refer to the guidelines I outlined on page 37 to help determine if a product is made from whole grains. Remember, finding a grain described as 100% whole grain in the ingredients list is more important than finding the words "whole grain" used loosely on the front of the package.

See pages 130–131 for my approved breads and cereals.

Watch Out for Corn

Many people who visit my office discover that they have a sensitivity to corn. I believe I'm seeing more people with corn sensitivity because a growing percentage of U.S. corn is genetically modified (as of 2004, 45 percent of all corn planted in the United States was genetically modified).[9] Therefore, I recommend that you limit your consumption of whole-grain products that contain corn.

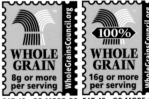

Sprouted Breads

I encourage you to go one step further than whole-wheat breads and eat sprouted breads and flat breads. Ezekiel bread and manna bread are both terrific flourless breads made from live, sprouted grains.

When you buy grain products, look for the word *sprouted* (as in "sprouted wheat") on the ingredient list.

Sprouted-grain products do go bad quicker, especially if you leave them on the counter, but there's nothing wrong with that. It means they aren't loaded with preservatives. The food God gave the Israelites during their sojourn in the wilderness—manna—bred worms after just one day. It's characteristic of live food.

Allergic to Wheat?

Millet bread and other millet products are a tasty, healthy alternative to whole-grain wheat products.

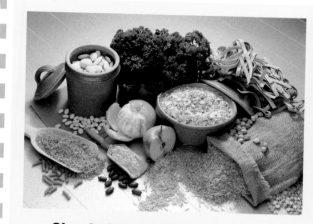

Simple Ways to "Hide" Whole Grains in Your Diet

- Add brown rice or rolled oats to recipes for meatballs, meatloaf, or hamburgers. A general rule of thumb: add ¾ cup of uncooked grains to every pound of meat.

- The next time you make cookies or muffins, try substituting half of the white flour with whole-wheat flour.

- Add ½ cup of cooked brown rice, wild rice, sorghum, or barley to your next batch of homemade or canned soup.

- Add ½ cup of cooked wild rice to your next batch of dressing or stuffing.

- Replace white rice with brown rice, basmati rice, or quinoa the next time you make risotto or rice pilaf.

- Sprinkle a handful of rolled oats on salad, yogurt, or ice cream.

- Use whole-grain pasta for your favorite pasta dishes.

- Blend your favorite ready-to-eat cereal with whole grains such as spelt or buckwheat.[10]

EAT MORE FIBER

I FREQUENTLY TREAT PEOPLE in my practice who tell me they have only one bowel movement a week and think that's normal. They're shocked when I tell them a healthy person should have a bowel movement after every meal. Every time you eat food, the colon should experience peristalsis, which is the gastrocolic reflex that propels food through your digestive system.

Inadequate intake of fiber is associated with increased constipation, hemorrhoids, diverticulosis, diverticulitis, bowel irregularities, and colorectal cancer. It is also associated

Food	Amount of Dietary Fiber
Pinto beans, ½ cup, cooked	7.4 grams
Artichoke, 1 medium, cooked	6.5 grams
Kidney beans, ½ cup, cooked	5.8 grams
Navy beans, ½ cup, cooked	5.8 grams
Apple, 3-inch diameter	5.7 grams
Figs, 3 small	5.3 grams
Orange, 3-inch diameter	4.4 grams
Green peas, ½ cup, cooked	4.3 grams
Raspberries, ½ cup	4.2 grams
Barley, ½ cup, cooked	4.2 grams
Blackberries, ½ cup	3.8 grams
Mango, medium	3.7 grams
Banana, 7 inches long	2.8 grams
Whole-wheat noodles, ½ cup	2.3 grams
Whole-wheat bread, 1 medium slice	1.9 grams
Brown rice, ½ cup, cooked	1.7 grams

Switch Slowly

When switching from a low-fiber diet to a high-fiber diet, do it in increments. If you do it too suddenly, you might experience bloating or gas.[11]

More Fiber Means More Water

Fiber and water work together to stimulate the colon. As you increase the amount of fiber in your diet, you should increase the amount of water you drink.

with elevated cholesterol, irritable bowel syndrome, toxin buildup, and poor blood sugar control in diabetics. Most Americans eat an estimated 12 grams or less of fiber daily. But the recommended goal is 25 to 30 grams a day.[12]

Dietary fiber is simply nondigestible polysaccharides, which are found in plant cell walls.[13] Many people get fiber from whole-grain cereals, nuts,

seeds, dried beans, fruits, and vegetables. Some other good sources are included in the table on page 58.[14]

There are two types of fiber: insoluble and soluble. Insoluble fiber increases the frequency of our bowel movements and the weight of our stool, and it helps prevent constipation, irritable bowel syndrome, hemorrhoids, diverticulosis, and other intestinal disorders. Bran (from any grain) is a good source of insoluble fiber. Most people can tolerate rice bran very well, so I often recommend this over the more

popular wheat bran. Other good sources are high-fiber cereals and the skins of vegetables and fruits.

Soluble fiber lowers cholesterol, stabilizes blood sugar, slows digestion, and helps your body bind and eliminate toxins. Good sources of soluble fiber include fruits, beans, legumes, lentils, carrots, oats, and seeds such as psyllium seed and flaxseed.

It's important to get both types of fiber in your diet. Generally speaking, the higher the fiber content of your foods, the better.

Quick Ways to Add More Fiber to Your Diet

- Add berries or almonds to your bowl of cereal or steel-cut oatmeal in the morning.
- Eat an orange or grapefruit instead of drinking a glass of juice. If you prefer drinking juice, squeeze your own and add the pulp back into the juice before drinking it.
- Sprinkle some pinto beans, garbanzo beans (chickpeas), or almonds on your salad.
- Switch to whole-grain pastas, cereals, and breads.
- Try the new double-fiber whole-grain breads.

Healthy Fats

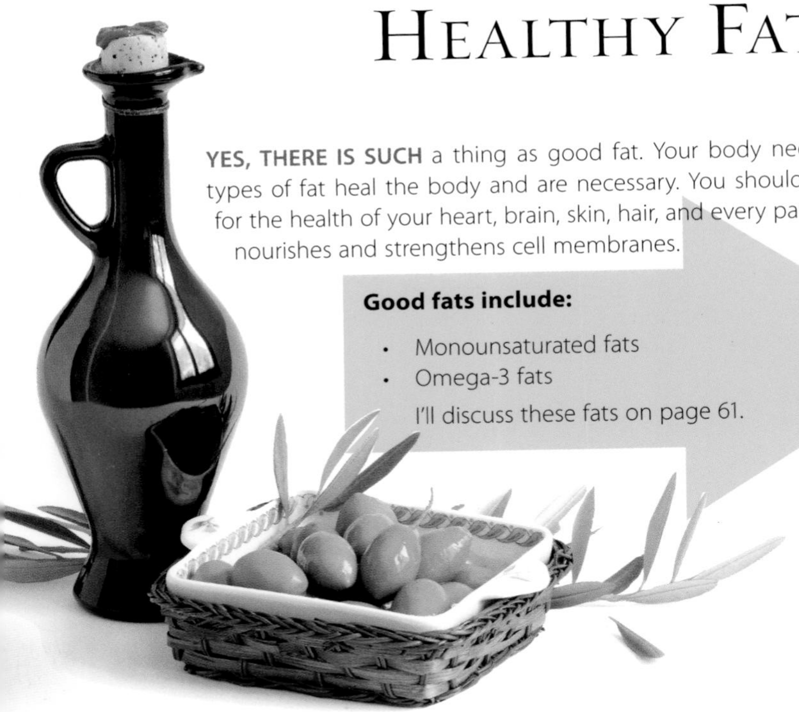

YES, THERE IS SUCH a thing as good fat. Your body needs fat! The good types of fat heal the body and are necessary. You should eat fat every day for the health of your heart, brain, skin, hair, and every part of you. Good fat nourishes and strengthens cell membranes.

Good fats include:

- Monounsaturated fats
- Omega-3 fats

I'll discuss these fats on page 61.

Dan's Famous Salad Dressing

My brother, Dan Colbert, has a wonderful recipe for healthy salad dressing. I like it so much that I share it often in my books and with my patients.

¼ cup balsamic vinegar

1 clove fresh garlic, minced

Pinch of sea salt

2 Tbsp. clean, pure water

Juice of one lemon

⅔ cup extra-virgin olive oil

Pour the balsamic vinegar into a glass salad dressing cruet (such as Good Seasons' mixing bottle), and add the remaining ingredients in the order listed. Refrigerate. Makes 1 cup.

TIP: Dressings prepared with olive oil may congeal when refrigerated. Let the refrigerated dressing reach room temperature before serving.

See pages 134–135 for all of the salad dressings, oils, and fats I recommend.

Monounsaturated fat is found in extra-virgin or virgin olive oil that is cold-pressed (not heated). You can also get monounsaturated fats in natural organic peanut butter, avocados, olives, macadamia nuts, and especially almonds, walnuts, and hazelnuts. Raw nuts and seeds—not the roasted, salted, flavored, and candied kind—should be a mainstay of your diet. I enjoy almonds, macadamia nuts, and walnuts. Almonds are excellent because they are high in monounsaturated fats and contain about 20 percent protein. Try almond butter.

Go easy with nuts and seeds at first, or you may upset your stomach. Start out light and gradually increase them. Remember, moderation is the key. Also, if you leave nuts unsealed for thirty days, they may become rancid, doing more harm than good. Keep nuts in #1 PETE plastic or ceramic containers, and place them in the refrigerator or freezer until you are ready to use them.

Omega-3 fatty acids are found mainly in cold-water fish, some marine mammals, and algae (seaweed). Scientists believe the best way to obtain adequate omega-3 is direct consumption of DHA (docosahexaenoic acid) and EPA (eicosapentaenoic acid) from fish. DHA protects the brain, reversing signs of brain aging and protecting against development of Alzheimer's and dementia. DHA also plays a role in preventing ADHD and impaired learning. EPA protects the heart and decreases inflammation. It has anticancer, anti-inflammatory, and anti-hypertensive effects. EPA reduces the risk of stroke, heart arrhythmias, dementia, and heart attack.[15]

Alpha-linolenic acid (ALA) is commonly lacking in the standard American diet. The fats in flaxseed, flaxseed oil, walnuts, and different green vegetables and super foods are converted in the body into ALA. The body then uses ALA to make EPA and DHA to nourish and protect the heart and brain and to produce a powerful hormone called "PG3," which reduces pain and inflammation and prevents platelets from adhering, which reduces blood clots.

Do You Need More ALA or Omega-3?

Unfortunately, many people are unable to convert ALA to omega-3. Therefore, rather than trying to increase your intake of ALA, concentrate on getting more omega-3 fats in your diet. I recommend that you eat wild salmon as a good source of omega-3 fats.

HEALTHY FATS
(CONTINUED)

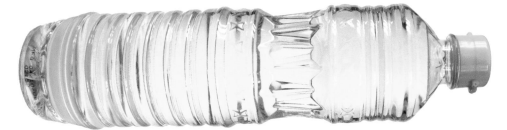

The canola controversy

Canola oil is a monounsaturated fat used primarily in cooking and food preparation. Although canola oil has been singled out by some nutritionists as having toxic properties, it

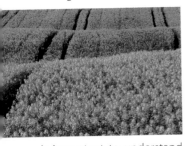

is important to understand that the nutritional value of any edible oil can be destroyed and turned into poison, depending on the processing and cooking techniques used. When canola was developed in the 1970s, oil from rapeseed, a member of the mustard family (pictured on this page), was used. Canola today has been hybridized from rapeseed to yield a good all-purpose cooking oil with high monounsaturated fat content similar to olive oil, but with a longer shelf life.

There has been concern over high levels of trans fatty acids, but canola oil that has not been hydrogenated will not have significant amounts of trans fats. It is important to check the label before purchasing. However, there still remains controversy. Dr. Mary Enig, PhD, one of the top biochemists in the country, found that canola oil has to be partially hydrogenated or refined before it is used commercially.[16]

The key to choosing a healthy oil is in the extraction process. Mass-market oils are usually chemically extracted from seeds using hexane, a petroleum product that is harmful to the environment and has the potential to leave a residue on the finished product.

Expeller pressing—and especially cold pressing—is a much healthier alternative for processing oils. In this process, an expeller press crushes seeds with hydraulic action. This process yields less oil than chemical extraction, which is why expeller-pressed oils are usually more expensive. Still, they are the best choice for cooking and eating.

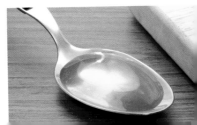

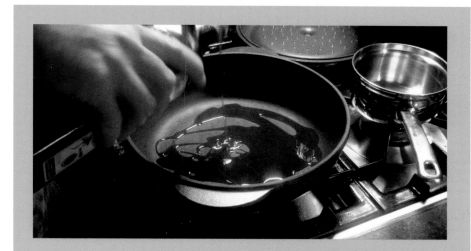

Choosing the Right Oil for the Job

If you enjoy fried foods, then switch to stir-frying, lightly, on low heat using organic extra-virgin coconut oil, organic butter, organic ghee (clarified butter), or organic macadamia nut oil, which has a fairly high smoke point. If you stir-fry with extra-virgin olive oil, do not stir-fry at high temperatures because it has a low smoke point. Never cook with flaxseed oil. *Smoke point* is the point at which the oil begins to break down, releasing free radicals. This may even occur at low temperatures. (See page 146 for more information.)

Avoid frying in polyunsaturated fats such as corn oil, sunflower oil, soybean oil, or safflower oil. Frying at high temperatures converts these oils to dangerous lipid peroxides, which create tremendous amounts of free radicals. These free radicals can damage the liver and cause chromosomal damage in lab animals. Imagine the amount of damage it is doing in our bodies, and especially in the bodies of our children as we continue to feed them french fries, fried chicken strips, and onion rings.

Most of the heat-processed oils go through various stages. Here is the process in a nutshell. The seed is heated to high temperatures (about 300 degrees Fahrenheit) and pressed to expel the oil; then the oil is degummed, which removes all of the valuable nutrients. At this point, the oil is heated again, but to 500 degrees Fahrenheit to remove the rancid odor and yellowish tinge. The end result is what you see on the grocery shelf—a clear, odorless oil full of lipid peroxides. See my book *What Would Jesus Eat?* for more information.[17]

ALKALINIZING FOODS

CELLS THRIVE IN AN alkaline environment but get constipated with metabolic waste and toxins in an acidic environment. To check the acidity of their bodies, I have my patients test their first morning urine pH, which is a good indicator of the pH of the tissues. For patients whose reading is below 7.0, I often recommend drinking fresh, juiced organic fruits and vegetables (which are sprouts and vegetables such as wheat grass, barley grass, oat grass, spirulina, chlorella, and blue green algae) or a phytonutrient powder drink to help cleanse and alkalinize the body as well as provide superior nutrition.

Your diet should probably consist of 50 percent (or higher) alkaline-forming foods and 50 percent (or less) acid-forming foods. That's about one serving of vegetables and one of fruit or other alkalinizing foods for every serving of acidic foods (meats or grains).

Alkaline-forming foods include most fruits, green vegetables, lentils, spices, herbs and seasonings, and seeds and nuts. Acid-forming foods include meat, fish, poultry, chicken eggs, most grains, legumes, and especially desserts, processed foods, and fast foods. Refer to the charts on these pages to help simplify it.[18]

ALKALIZING FOODS	
Vegetables	Alfalfa • Barley grass • Beets • Broccoli • Cabbage • Carrots • Cauliflower •Celery • Chlorella • Collard greens • Cucumber • Eggplant • Garlic • Green beans • Green peas • Kale • Lettuce • Mushrooms • Mustard greens • Nightshade veggies • Onions • Peas • Peppers • Pumpkin • Radishes • Rutabaga • Spinach, green • Sprouts • Sweet potatoes • Tomatoes • Watercress • Wild greens • Wheat grass
Fruits	Apple • Apricot • Avocado • Banana • Berries • Blackberries • Blueberries • Cantaloupe • Cherries, sour • Coconut, fresh • Cranberries • Currants • Dates, dried • Figs, dried • Grapes • Grapefruit • Honeydew melon • Lemon • Lime • Muskmelons • Nectarine • Orange • Peach • Pear • Pineapple • Raisins • Raspberries • Strawberries • Tangerine • Tomato • Tropical fruits • Watermelon
Grains	Millet
Nuts	Almonds • Chestnuts
Sweeteners	Stevia
Spices and Seasonings	Chili pepper • Cinnamon • Curry • Ginger • Herbs (all) • Mustard • Sea salt
Other	Alkaline antioxidant water • Apple cider vinegar • Duck eggs • Fresh, squeezed fruit juice • Ghee (clarified butter) • Green juices • Mineral water • Quail eggs • Soured dairy products • Veggie juices
Minerals	Calcium: pH 12 • Cesium: pH 14 • Magnesium: pH 9 • Potassium: pH 14 • Sodium: pH 14

ACIDIFYING FOODS	
Vegetables	Corn • Olives • Winter squash
Fruits	Pickled fruits • Cranberries
Grains, Grain Products	Barley • Bran, oat • Bran, wheat • Bread • Corn • Cornstarch • Crackers, soda • Flour, wheat • Flour, white • Macaroni • Noodles • Rice (all) • Rice cakes • Rye • Spaghetti • Spelt • Wheat germ • Wheat
Beans and Legumes	Black beans • Chick peas • Kidney beans • Lima beans • Pinto beans • Soybeans • White beans
Dairy	Butter • Cheese • Cheese, processed • Ice cream • Ice milk
Nuts and Butters	Brazil nuts • Hazelnuts • Legumes • Peanut butter • Peanuts • Pecans • Pine nuts • Walnuts
Animal Protein	Bacon • Beef • Carp • Clams • Cod • Corned beef • Fish • Haddock • Lamb • Lobster • Mussels • Organ meats • Oyster • Pike • Pork • Rabbit • Salmon • Sardines • Sausage • Scallops • Shellfish • Shrimp • Tuna • Turkey • Veal • Venison
Fats and Oils	Almond oil • Butter • Canola oil • Corn oil • Safflower oil • Sesame oil • Sunflower oil • All fried foods
Sweeteners	Corn syrup • Sugar
Other Foods	Catsup • Cocoa • Coffee • Mustard • Pepper • Soft drinks • Vinegar
Drugs and Chemicals	Aspirin • Chemicals • Drugs, medicinal • Drugs, psychedelic • Herbicides • Pesticides • Tobacco

Acid Test

If you would like to know how acidic your body is, buy pH strips at the drugstore. Collect your first morning urine and dip pH paper into it. It will indicate your urine's pH level with a change of color. The change of color can then be matched to a numerical reading. A card is included in the pH paper that correlates a color to a pH number. It is similar to checking the pH of a swimming pool.

Your pH test reading should be between 7.0 to 7.5. It may take you a while to achieve this pH, but keep at it. Drink alkaline water and eat alkaline foods (such as fruits and vegetables).

The Benefits of Alkaline Water

Clean, alkaline water unburdens your liver and kidneys. It also supports your colon, enabling it to work as it should. Like alkalinizing foods, alkaline water also helps alkalinize your tissues, another important step in balancing your body for optimal health.

THE POWER OF PHYTONUTRIENTS

LIVING FOODS ARE POWERFUL sources of one of the major ingredients for optimum health: phytonutrients. Phytonutrients are biologically active substances that give fruits and vegetables their color, flavor, smell, and natural disease resistance. They can have major health benefits for your body, which I will cover on the next several pages.

Some researchers estimate forty thousand phytonutrients will one day be catalogued and understood.[19] At the present time, there are over two thousand known phytonutrients. These compounds protect plants from pests, excessive amounts of ultraviolet radiation, and disease. Each plant has thousands of different phytonutrients that provide protection from free radicals because they contain natural antioxidants.

In humans, phytonutrient consumption is associated with reduced rates of many different cancers. They also protect against heart disease and protect or slow the progression of dementia and age-related cognitive decline. They increase longevity, are associated with reduced rates of chronic disease, and protect us against cataracts and macular degeneration. Phytonutrients are hard at work in your body, saving you from various threats of which you likely are never aware.

Blueberries

Blueberries contain polyphenols that protect the brain from inflammation and oxidative stress, which in turn may protect the brain from the degenerative effects of aging and from injury from ischemic stroke.[20] Blueberries may even help prevent Alzheimer's disease and Parkinson's disease. When rats suffering from Alzheimer's-like symptoms were supplemented with blueberries in their diets, they were able to perform normally on tests involving memory and motor behavior.[21] I recommend a serving of organic blueberries every day.

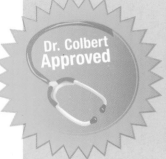
Dr. Colbert Approved

ORAC Scores for Produce

One way to judge the benefits of each fruit and vegetable is by their Oxygen Radical Absorbance Capacity, or ORAC. This is a standard tool used by nutritionists to measure foods' antioxidant capacity. The higher the ORAC, the higher the concentration of antioxidants in that food, and the greater protection it provides against free radicals.

It seems that every time I turn around, a different food has been ranked as number one—I've seen blueberries, cranberries, acai, and even Granny Smith apples all given the honor of top antioxidant billing, depending on the source of information. Perhaps you've noticed this too and are wondering how it happens. It depends on a few variables in the ranking process:

1. Did they use ORAC or a different test such as FRAP (Ferric Reducing Ability of Plasma) to measure the antioxidant levels of foods?
2. Did they single out specific categories of foods (such as fruits and vegetables) for comparison, or are all foods included?
3. Did they compare average serving sizes or use a gram-per-gram comparison?

I believe we will continue to see changing ORAC rankings for foods because new fruits and other edible plants are still being discovered in the Amazon rainforest and other places. This is why acai has recently topped the charts but doesn't appear on older ORAC listings. In the future, as these new foods are tested, they will likely prove to have even higher ORAC scores.

Regardless of whether your favorite foods receive top billing or not, as long as they consistently show up somewhere on the ORAC report card, you can rest assured that they are helping your body fight free radicals when you eat them. Here's the way fruits and vegetables were ranked in a comprehensive ORAC report done by the USDA in 2004:[22]

Top-Scoring Fruits & Vegetables

Fruits	ORAC units per 100 grams	Vegetables	ORAC units per 100 grams
Prunes	5,770	Kale	1,770
Raisins	2,830	Spinach	1,260
Blueberries	2,400	Brussels sprouts	980
Blackberries	2,036	Alfalfa sprouts	930
Strawberries	1,540	Broccoli flowers	890
Raspberries	1,220	Beets	840
Plums	949	Red bell pepper	710
Oranges	750	Onion	450
Red grapes	739	Corn	400
Cherries	670	Eggplant	390

PHYTONUTRIENTS: A RAINBOW OF HEALTH

THE PHYTONUTRIENTS IN FRUITS and vegetables can be grouped according to color. Each group has its own set of unique protective benefits. You need to try to consume all seven colors of the phytonutrient rainbow every day to receive the protection you need. To do this, you need to eat a variety of foods. Think of phytonutrients as a "rainbow of health," God's promise to you to keep you healthy. Let's look at each group.

Classes of Phytonutrients

Typically, phytonutrients are classified by their chemical structures. This is an extensive classification, and it is also quite confusing, since many phytonutrients provide similar protection. The main classifications include:

- *Organo-sulfurs*, such as cruciferous vegetables and the sulfur compound in garlic

- *Terpenoids*, such as limonene in citrus as well as carotenoids, tocopherols, tocotrienols, etc.

- *Flavonoids*, including certain red/purple pigmented fruits and vegetables

- *Isoflavonoids* and *lignans* found in soy foods and flaxseeds

- *Organic acids* found in whole grains, parsley, licorice, and citrus fruits

Since there are so many different phytonutrients, they are also classified in families, and this depends on the similarities in their structure. As you can see, it can be quite confusing! That's why I like to simply group them by color.

EAT THIS AND LIVE!

Red

Tomatoes, watermelon, guava, and red grapefruit contain a powerful carotenoid called *lycopene*, which is about twice as powerful as beta-carotene. Lycopene is the main pigment responsible for the red color. Lycopene is linked to prevention of heart disease and prostate cancer. A study conducted by Harvard researchers examined the relationship between carotenoids and the risk of prostate cancer. Only the carotenoid lycopene was associated with protection. The men in this study with the greatest protection against prostate cancer consumed at least 6.5 mg a day of lycopene from tomato products.[23]

Orange

Orange-colored fruits and vegetables, including carrots, mangoes, cantaloupes, pumpkin, sweet potatoes, yams, squash, and apricots, have high amounts of carotenoids, which help prevent cancer and heart disease. Typically, the more orange the fruit or vegetable is, the higher the concentration of *provitamin A carotenoids* (carotenoids that can be transformed into vitamin A). Orange fruits and vegetables generally are also high in *beta-carotene*. Eating just one small carrot every day may help protect you from cancer.[24]

Red/Purple

Blueberries, blackberries, hawthorn berries, raspberries, grapes, eggplants, red cabbage, and red wine contain a powerful flavonoid called *anthocyanidin*, which contains approximately fifty times the antioxidant activity of vitamin C and is twenty times more powerful than vitamin E.

Pine bark, grape seeds and skins, bilberry, and cranberry contain another flavonoid, *proanthocyanidin*, which helps maintain the elasticity in our skin and blood vessels, preventing wrinkles, spider veins, and varicose veins.

Resveratrol is found in red grape skins and seeds, purple grape juice, and red wine; it helps prevent the progression of cancer, prevents blood clots, raises HDL or "good" cholesterol, and promotes longevity.

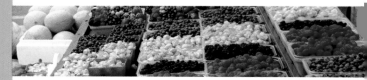

Orange/Yellow

Oranges, tangerines, lemons, limes, yellow grapefruit, papaya, pineapple, and nectarines are rich in vitamin C and *citrus bioflavonoids* and protect us against free-radical damage. Citrus bioflavonoids increase intracellular levels of vitamin C, strengthen blood vessels, and maintain the collagen that forms tendons, cartilage, and ligaments. They prevent allergies and inflammation and have also been used to prevent and treat bruising, hemorrhoids, varicose veins, and spider veins.

Yellow/Green

Spinach, kale, collard greens, mustard greens, turnip greens, romaine lettuce, leeks, and peas are typically rich in *lutein* and *zeaxanthin*. Lutein is able to reduce the risk of macular degeneration, which is the leading cause of blindness in older adults. One study found that adults with the highest dietary intake of lutein had a 57 percent lower risk of macular degeneration than individuals with the lowest intake.[25] Lutein may also protect the lens of the eye from sunlight damage, slowing down the development of cataracts.

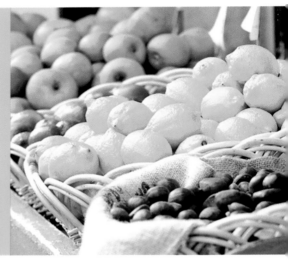

Green

Broccoli, cabbage, brussels sprouts, cauliflower, watercress, bok choy, kale, collard greens, and mustard greens are considered cruciferous vegetables. These cancer fighters contain more phytonutrients with anticancer properties than any other family of vegetables.

Studies have correlated a high intake of cruciferous vegetables, especially cabbage, with lower rates of cancers of the breast, prostate, and colon. Broccoli sprouts have some of the highest concentration of protective phytonutrients. Young broccoli sprouts that are about three days old contain twenty to fifty times more phytonutrients than mature broccoli.

White/Green

Onions and garlic contain powerful phytonutrients. Onions contain the flavonoid *quercetin*, which has anti-inflammatory, antiviral, and anticancer properties. Quercetin is often recommended by nutritionists to treat both allergies and asthma. Apples, red wine, and black tea also contain quercetin.

Several of the components in garlic have significant anticancer effects. Garlic also inhibits the formation of *nitrosamines*, which are cancer-causing compounds formed during digestion. Garlic has significant antimicrobial activity against bacteria, viruses, fungi, and even parasites. It also has cholesterol-lowering activities and can even lower blood pressure as well as help prevent blood clots.

Green tea's active constituents are *polyphenols*, which have been shown to reduce the risk of cancers of the stomach, small intestines, colon, and pancreas, as well as lung and breast cancers. As an antioxidant, green tea is two hundred times more powerful than vitamin E and five hundred times more powerful than vitamin C. It provides powerful antioxidants to help repair damaged DNA. It also activates detoxification enzymes in the liver, which helps defend your body against cancer. The normal amount of green tea consumed by the Japanese is about three cups a day.

I also recommend organic white tea, which I discuss more on page 106.

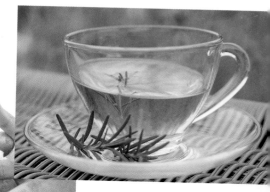

FRUITS AND VEGETABLES

HALF OF YOUR DIET should be raw, organic fruits and vegetables and whole grains. Even adding one serving a day can lower your heart disease risk. A serving size of fruits and vegetables is typically ½ cup to 1 cup, which is 4 to 8 ounces. When in doubt, I tell people to picture the size of a tennis ball. A diet rich in fruits and vegetables can often reduce blood pressure as much as medication does. People who eat more than four servings a day have lower levels of bad cholesterol. Studies clearly show that for preventing cancer, fruits and vegetables are the best "medicine." The natural phytonutrients in produce protect against all kinds of cancer.[26] In this chapter I've covered the importance of eating a wide variety of fruits and vegetables. Here are a few final suggestions:

- Eat plenty of nonstarchy vegetables like spinach, lettuce, cabbage, broccoli, asparagus, green beans, radishes, turnips, and cauliflower.

- Starchy vegetables like beans, peas, potatoes, and sweet potatoes are fine in moderation.

- Eat colorful salads with balsamic or red wine vinegar and extra-virgin olive oil or other healthy oils from the good fats previously discussed.

The New Super Berry: Acai

The acai berry is gaining in popularity daily, largely because word is spreading that it is rich in antioxidants like vitamin A, vitamin C, and calcium. It is also a good source of omega-3s, fiber, protein, carbohydrates, and minerals. But topping the headlines is a report published in the *Journal of Agriculture and Food Chemistry* in 2007, which stated that of all fruits and vegetables tested to date, freeze-dried acai, with a score of 1,614 units/g, had the highest activity against superoxide in the superoxide scavenging (SOD) assay.[27]

Cancer-Preventing Broccoli Sprouts

In 1997, scientists from Johns Hopkins discovered that three-day-old broccoli sprouts—which look and taste similar to alfalfa sprouts—contain 20 to 50 times the amount of sulforaphane found in mature broccoli. *Sulforaphane* is a compound discovered in 1992 that helps your body arm itself against cancer. It has been suggested that eating a few tablespoons of sprouts a day can provide your body with the same amount of chemoprotection as eating one to two pounds of broccoli a week.[28]

For this reason, I've started growing my own broccoli sprouts at home, and I recommend this practice to my patients as well. Sprouting kits can be found at most health foods stores and online.

EAT THIS AND LIVE!

Pomegranate Power

Research continually shows the benefits of pomegranate—one of the world's richest sources of antioxidants. Pomegranate protects your heart by protecting arterial walls and improving blood flow to the heart.

Studies also show that pomegranate helps arm your body against cardiovascular disease inhibiting the oxidation of LDL (bad) cholesterol.

In addition, pomegranate may reverse atherosclerosis. In a recent study, Israeli scientists found that among patients given daily pomegranate supplements, lesions in the carotid artery decreased in size by 35 percent. The lesions in those who did not take pomegranate actually grew by 9 percent. This means that pomegranate reversed existing atherosclerosis.

The same Israeli scientists found that drinking as little as 2 ounces of pomegranate juice a day was shown to reduce blood pressure.

In addition to its heart-healthy benefits, pomegranate may help people with diabetes and pre-diabetes by lowering after-meal blood sugar levels.

It is also shown to halt the progression of prostate cancer in men who had undergone surgery or radiation for the disease.

As if that's not enough, it is also possible that pomegranate may fight the degeneration of joint tissue that leads to osteoarthritis and may protect the brain against Alzheimer's disease.[29]

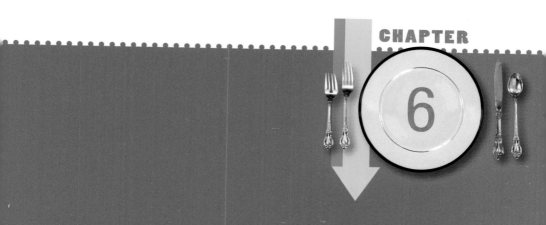

TARGETING YOUR INTAKE OF SPECIFIC ANTIOXIDANTS, VITAMINS, AND MINERALS

ANTIOXIDANTS, VITAMINS, AND MINERALS

TO UNDERSTAND THE IMPORTANCE of antioxidants, you must first understand free radicals. So, exactly what is a free radical? Picture an atom that has a nucleus with pairs of electrons circling around it. When an electron becomes unpaired, it tries to pull an electron from another atom or molecule to return to a state of equilibrium. Free radicals are simply atoms with unpaired electrons. As they steal electrons from other atoms, they cause a chain reaction of cell damage.

Many diseases create tremendous amounts of free radicals, including most cancers, arthritis, coronary artery disease, asthma, Alzheimer's disease, Parkinson's disease, multiple sclerosis, lupus, and colitis. Frequent colds, flu, sinus infections, bronchitis, and bladder and yeast infections create more free radicals. Trauma from sprains, strains, and muscle aches also add to the amount of free radicals in the body.

But these aren't the only ways that free radicals are produced. Free radicals are generated in our bodies simply by breathing! Normal metabolism creates millions of free radicals referred to as reactive oxygen species (ROS) in our bodies every day. Eating dead foods—including unhealthy fats, highly processed foods, high-sugar foods, fried foods, sauces, gravies, and so on—laced with chemicals and pesticides produces excessive amounts of free radicals that cause disease, which creates even more free radicals.

The way to keep these free radicals at bay is simple: antioxidants. Antioxidants have the ability to neutralize free radicals. Antioxidants are to free radicals what water is to a raging forest fire burning out of control.

Different antioxidants are able to neutralize free radicals in every part of the body. I believe that it's important to take supplements of key antioxidants, and I explain these in my book *The Seven Pillars of Health*. It's also important to fortify your body by eating foods that provide a wide variety of antioxidants. On the facing page is a list of the top twenty antioxidant foods you should make a regular part of your diet.

Vitamins and minerals

Most people have the misconception that vitamins will give them instant energy. Vitamins are not pep pills; *vitamin* literally means "vital amine," and they are indeed needed for many biological processes, including growth, digestion, mental alertness, and resistance to infection. Vitamins enable your body to use carbohydrates, fats, and proteins, and they speed up chemical reactions. Vitamins and minerals are not optional for your health. They are at the very foundation of your health.

Most Americans don't get even basic amounts of recommended vitamins and minerals. On the next four pages, I will give you some fast facts on the vitamins and minerals most Americans lack, what those nutrients do, the foods in which they are found, and what happens when you don't get enough of them.

EAT THIS AND LIVE!

Top Twenty Antioxidant Foods

A terrific study in the June 2004 issue of the *Journal of Agriculture and Food Chemistry* tested the antioxidant power of more than one hundred different kinds of fruits, vegetables, nuts, and spices. They came up with a list of the top antioxidant foods. The top twenty are:[1]

1. Mexican red beans (dried)
2. Wild blueberries
3. Red kidney beans
4. Pinto beans
5. Cultivated blueberries
6. Cranberries
7. Artichokes (cooked)
8. Blackberries
9. Prunes
10. Raspberries
11. Strawberries
12. Red Delicious apples
13. Granny Smith apples
14. Pecans
15. Cherries
16. Black plums
17. Russet potatoes (cooked)
18. Black beans (dried)
19. Red plums
20. Gala apples

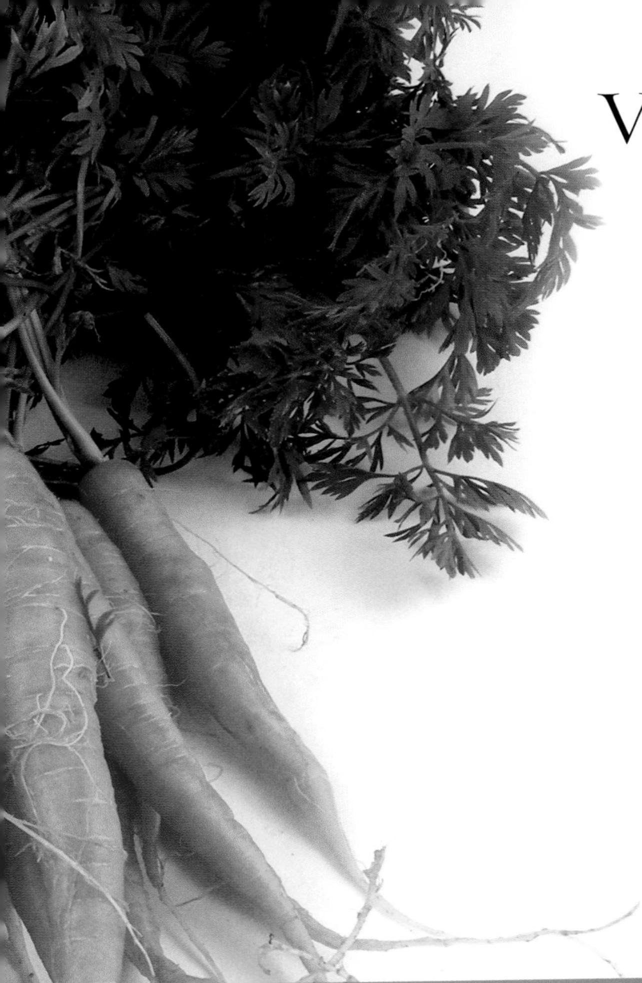

VITAMIN A

AN ESTIMATED 44 PERCENT of Americans are lacking adequate intake of vitamin A,[2] which protects us against cancer and heart disease, prevents night blindness and other eye problems, helps the skin repair itself, and helps in the formation of bones and teeth. Vitamin A (retinol) is important for the immune system, protecting us against colds, the flu, and infections of the kidneys, bladder, lungs, and mucous membranes.

Beta-carotene is converted in the body to vitamin A. The recommended daily intake (RDI) for most adults is 2,300 to 3,000 IU (international units) daily. Lactating women need 4,000 IU a day. Children need only 1,000 to 2,000 IU daily.[3]

The chart below gives some food sources for vitamin A and beta-carotene:[4]

Sources of Vitamin A		Sources of Beta-Carotene	
Food	Amount of Vitamin A	Food	Amount of Beta-Carotene
Cod liver oil, 1 tsp.	2,000 IU	Carrots, boiled, ½ cup slices	13,418 IU
Milk, fortified skim, 1 cup	500 IU	Carrot, raw, 7 inches	8,666 IU
Cheese, cheddar, 1 oz.	249 IU	Cantaloupe, cubed, 1 cup	5,411 IU
		Spinach, raw, 1 cup	2,813 IU
		Mango, sliced, 1 cup	1,262 IU
		Peach, 1 medium	319 IU

Want to Live to Be 100?

Blood levels of antioxidants generally decrease with age. However, Italian researchers discovered that centenarians (people one hundred years of age or older) needed significantly higher blood levels of vitamin A and vitamin E than their younger counterparts. The researchers concluded that these two vitamins seem to be very important in guaranteeing longevity.[5]

EAT THIS AND LIVE!

Vitamin A Deficiency

Lack of vitamin A in your body can cause dry hair and skin, dry eyes, poor growth, frequent colds, skin disorders, sinusitis, insomnia, fatigue, and respiratory infections.[6]

Caution

Be careful not to go overboard when taking vitamin A because excessive amounts of vitamin A may lead to liver damage.[7] Dosages greater than 10,000 IU a day of vitamin A were reported in the *New England Journal of Medicine* to have probably been responsible for one out of fifty-seven birth defects in the United States. However, this does not refer to beta-carotene or other carotenoids.[8] Women who are at risk for becoming pregnant should keep their supplemental vitamin A levels below 5,000 IU or choose carotenoids instead of vitamin A.[9] Also, carotenoids, such as beta-carotene, are safer than vitamin A because the body will convert beta-carotene to vitamin A without producing vitamin A in toxic amounts.[10]

VITAMIN B₆

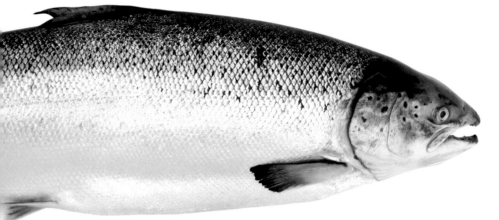

VITAMIN B₆ (PYRIDOXINE) PERFORMS many functions in your body, but studies show that 28 percent of women nineteen years of age and older do not have adequate intake of this vitamin.[11] It is needed for more than one hundred enzymes involved in protein metabolism; it is also essential for red blood cell metabolism. The nervous and immune systems need it to function efficiently. It helps increase the amount of oxygen carried to your tissues, and it helps to keep your blood sugar level in a normal range. It is very important in the synthesis of neurotransmitters—serotonin and dopamine.[12]

Vitamin B₆ is found in fortified cereals, fish, poultry, red meat, and some produce. Recommended intake for adults age nineteen to fifty is 1.3 mg a day, and around 1.6 mg for people over fifty.[13]

Food	Amount of Vitamin B₆
Potato, medium, baked	0.70 mg
Banana, medium	0.68 mg
Chicken, ½ breast, cooked	0.52 mg
Garlic, 1 oz.	0.35 mg
Brussels sprouts, 1 cup, boiled	0.28 mg
Collard greens, 1 cup, drained, boiled	0.24 mg
Sunflower seeds, kernels only, 1 oz., dry roasted	0.23 mg
Red bell peppers, 1 cup, sliced, raw	0.23 mg
Broccoli pieces, 1 cup, steamed	0.22 mg
Watermelon, 1 cup	0.22 mg
Tomato juice, 6 oz.	0.20 mg
Avocado, raw, ½ cup, sliced	0.20 mg

Too Much of a Good Thing

If you take vitamin supplements, beware. Like anything else in life, too much of a good thing may eventually harm your body. Megadosing on one type of vitamin or mineral is no different. For example, megadoses of vitamin B_6 can lead to neuropathy or damage to nerves in your arms and legs.[14]

Vitamin B_6 Deficiency

Signs of vitamin B_6 deficiency include skin irritation, headaches, sore tongue, depression, confusion, convulsions, anemia, and PMS. If you are deficient in vitamin B_6, B_{12}, or folic acid, then levels of homocysteine, a toxic amino acid, may rise in the blood. Homocysteine has a toxic effect on the cells lining the arteries, causing plaque to form on the artery lining. High levels of homocysteine in the blood are associated with increased risk of cardiovascular disease as well as Alzheimer's disease.[15]

VITAMIN C

VITAMIN C IS AN antioxidant found in both plants and animals. Vitamin C (ascorbic acid) helps form collagen, a protein that gives structure to—and maintains—bones, cartilage, muscle, and blood vessels. It also plays a role in wound healing. The adequate intake is 90 mg per day for adult men and 75 mg for adult women, but studies show that 31 percent of Americans don't get enough.[16] Common sources include:[17]

Food	Amount of Vitamin C
Guava, 1 medium	165 mg
Red bell pepper, ½ cup	95 mg
Papaya, 1 medium	95 mg
Orange, 1 medium	60 mg
Broccoli, ½ cup, steamed	60 mg
Strawberries, ½ cup	45 mg
Cantaloupe, ½ cup	35 mg

The Fab Five

The five most important antioxidants, according to Lester Packer, PhD, professor of molecular and cell biology at the University of California and author of the book *The Antioxidant Miracle*, include vitamin C, vitamin E, coenzyme Q_{10}, alpha-lipoic acid, and glutathione.[18]

EAT THIS and LIVE!

Vitamin C Deficiency

Vitamin C deficiency causes weakness, fatigue, swollen gums, nosebleeds, and, in extreme cases, scurvy.[19] During stress, there are higher requirements for vitamin C. It is also reported to reduce the risk of cataracts and retinal damage, increase immune function, and decrease heavy metal toxicity. Increased intake of vitamin C is linked to a reduced risk of cancer of the cervix, stomach, colon, and lungs. It also reduces LDL oxidation, which causes plaque buildup in arteries, and it supports healthy blood pressure.[20]

Supplements: Easy Does It

Taking vitamin supplements with massive amounts of vitamin C, as was the fad in past decades, may cause kidney stones.[21] Also, nutrients work synergistically; simply supplementing one vitamin or mineral may cause imbalances in another vitamin or mineral. That's one of the reasons why, even though I recommend taking supplements, I also stress that your primary source of vitamins and minerals should be a balanced diet.

VITAMIN D

RESEARCH INDICATES THAT 20 percent of children and adults up to age fifty and 95 percent of adults over fifty do not have adequate intake of vitamin D (calciferol),[22] which is required for your body to absorb calcium and phosphorus. It is critically important for growth and for the normal development of bones and teeth.[23] It may protect against prostate and breast cancer and help prevent autoimmune diseases such as multiple sclerosis. The higher the vitamin D levels in the blood, the lower the risk for colon and colorectal cancers.[24]

Sun exposure is the most important source of vitamin D, because the skin synthesizes vitamin D in response to UV rays. Most people need only ten to fifteen minutes of direct sun exposure, twice a week, without sunscreen, to meet their vitamin D requirement.[25] However, few doctors recommend this since it may increase the risk of skin cancer for some individuals.

There are few good dietary sources of vitamin D. Cod liver oil offers a whopping 1,360 IU per tablespoon. I typically don't recommend cod liver oil because it usually contains many toxins. It also has to be overprocessed, thus rendering it unstable, and it contains a high percentage of oxidized fats. Three and one-half ounces of cooked salmon gives 360 IUs of vitamin D. And a cup of milk fortified with vitamin D gives about 100 IU.[26]

Vitamin D_3 is the active form of vitamin D. In its active form, vitamin D enhances the absorption of calcium from the small intestines. Even though the recommended dose of vitamin D for adults over fifty is 400–600 IU a day, the National Osteoporosis Foundation recommends 800 IU for those at risk.[27]

Gonna Soak Up Some Sun:

If you don't have a history of skin or pre-skin cancer, consider spending five to ten minutes a day in sunlight without sunblock. This enables your body to produce adequate amounts of vitamin D. Don't forget to wear sunglasses!

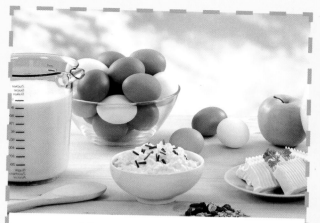

Vitamin D Deficiency

Vitamin D deficiency is common among young women (only 20 to 40 percent get the amounts they need) and in people over fifty, particularly women, for whom vitamin D deficiency is epidemic.[28] Many of my patients have such low levels of vitamin D in their blood that I typically will recommend 2,000 to 4,000 IU a day based on their blood levels of vitamin D.

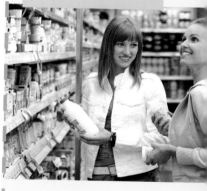

Vitamin D deficiency is associated with osteoporosis and hip fractures. In a review of women with osteoporosis, hospitalized for hip fractures, 50 percent were found to have signs of vitamin D deficiency.[29]

Too Much Vitamin D

Taking too much vitamin D can cause:

- Nausea
- Constipation
- Weight Loss
- Confusion[30]

New Vitamin D Requirements for Kids

In October 2008, the American Academy of Pediatrics released new guidelines recommending a daily dose of 400 IUs of vitamin D per child due to reports that rickets may be on the rise in the United States. Since most infants and young children will not consume the six glasses of milk or servings of salmon or mackerel that would provide them with 400 IUs of vitamin D, pediatricians expect most parents to meet the new guidelines by providing supplements for their children.[31]

VITAMIN E

RESEARCH SHOWS THAT 93 percent of Americans have inadequate intakes of vitamin E,[32] an antioxidant that decreases free-radical damage of lipid membranes and protects the heart, blood vessels, and tissues of the breast, liver, eyes, skin, and testes. Vitamin E (tocopherols, tocotrienols) decreases blood clotting, which further reduces the risk of heart disease.

Most people get vitamin E from vegetable oil products like salad dressings, though cold-pressed vegetables (such as extra-virgin olive oil) are generally highest in vitamin E. (Most vegetable oils are heat processed.) You can also get vitamin E from dark green leafy vegetables, legumes, nuts, seeds, whole grains, brown rice, corn meal, eggs, milk, oatmeal, and wheat germ. Common sources include the following:[33]

Food	Amount of Vitamin E
Wheat germ oil, 1 Tbsp.	20.3 mg (about 30 IU*)
Almonds, dried, 1 oz.	6.72 mg (about 10 IU)
Sweet potato, 1 medium	5.93 mg (about 9 IU)
* An IU (International Unit) is a unit of measurement used in pharmacology based on the biological activity of the substance being measured.	

Protection Against Prostate Cancer

One form of vitamin E, gamma-tocopherol, is extremely important. One study found that men with the highest concentration of gamma-tocopherol had a fivefold lower risk of developing prostate cancer than men with the lowest levels.[34] Gamma-tocopherol may also protect one from developing colorectal cancer and Alzheimer's disease.

Vitamin E Controversy

Tremendous confusion and even controversy have surrounded vitamin E since its discovery in 1922. One recent study concluded that in patients with vascular disease or diabetes, long-term supplementation with the natural source of vitamin E (400 IU) does not prevent cancer or cardiovascular events and may actually increase the risk for heart failure.[36] That conclusion had unfortunate consequences, because most Americans already lack sufficient amounts of this important nutrient. Some doctors warned their patients not to take vitamin E in a supplement.

The study also ignored the benefits of vitamin E. A different study showed that men who take 50 IU a day, as opposed to the recommended daily value of 30 IU, had 41 percent fewer deaths from prostate cancer than those who did not receive supplemental vitamin E.[37] That's a significant benefit.

Vitamin E Deficiency

Prolonged vitamin E deficiency may eventually cause severe neurological complications, including unsteady gait, loss of muscle coordination, muscle weakness, peripheral neuropathy, and diminished reflexes. It can also cause infertility, menstrual problems, miscarriages, and shortened red blood cell life span.

Natural vs. Synthetic

I recommend natural vitamin E, which should contain all eight forms of vitamin E: alpha-, beta-, delta-, and gamma-tocopherol, and alpha-, beta-, delta-, and gamma-tocotrienol. The names of all types of vitamin E begin with either "d" or "dl." The "d" is the natural form, and the "dl" is the synthetic form, which comes from petroleum. The synthetic form has only about 50 percent of the activity of natural vitamin E.[35]

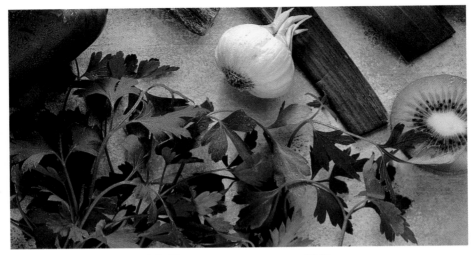

VITAMIN K

VITAMIN K IS A family of vitamins first identified in the 1920s and named with a K because of their importance in blood clotting, also called *coagulation* (*K* for koagulation). Vitamin K_1 is found in plants, and vitamin K_2 is primarily produced by bacteria in the intestines—including probiotic bacteria ("good" bacteria). The body can store about a one-month supply of the vitamin.

While vitamin K's role in blood clotting has been known for decades, its importance in regulating the function of calcium has only recently been recognized. Vitamin K_1 and, more importantly, vitamin K_2, play critical roles in preventing arterial calcification. So, exactly what is arterial calcification? Allow me to explain.

By now you are aware that as you age, you run the risk of losing calcium from your bones and developing osteopenia or osteoarthritis. But you may not know that as you lose calcium from your bones and teeth, your body actually deposits calcium in your arterial walls and heart valves, and the plaque in your arteries begins to resemble bone. This is arterial calcification.

Food Sources of Vitamin K

Studies suggest that 73 percent of Americans do not get adequate intake of vitamin K.[38] The daily reference intake for vitamin K for men age nineteen and above is 120 mcg (micrograms). For women in that age bracket it is 90 mcg.[39] Vitamin K (phylloquinone) is found in:[40]

Food	Amount of Vitamin K
Brussels sprouts, 1 cup, cooked	460 mcg
Broccoli, 1 cup, cooked	248 mcg
Cauliflower, 1 cup, cooked	150 mcg
Swiss chard, 1 cup, cooked	123 mcg
Spinach, 1 cup, raw	120 mcg
Beef, 3.5 oz.	104 mcg

You also may not realize that this is not a universal problem all people face as they age. While this is common in America, most elderly people in China and Japan have strong bones and teeth as well as clean, flexible, elastic arteries free of calcified plaque.

So, why is it that most aging Americans suffer from slowly melting bones and hardening, calcified arteries? The reason is simple: most of us lack vitamin K_2 in our diets. The Rotterdam Heart Study, which tracked 4,800 people for seven years, revealed that individuals who consumed the largest amounts of vitamin K_2 in their diet had a 57 percent reduction in death from heart disease than those who ingested the least. Also, individuals who ingested larger quantities had less calcium deposits in the aorta. However, those who consumed significantly less K_2 were more likely to develop moderate to severe calcification. Participants who consumed over 32.7 mcg a day in their diet had the lowest risk of heart attack and calcification of the aorta.[41]

Vitamin K_2's job is to make sure calcium gets to the right places and keep it from being deposited in the wrong places. The right places include the bones and blood. The wrong places include bone spurs and calcification of the arteries and soft tissues.

The food that is the richest source of vitamin K_2 is soy natto, which is a staple of the diet of many Japanese people. Vitamin K_2 is also found in much smaller amounts in egg yolks, fermented cheeses (not processed cheese), and organ meats, which I do not recommend. Vitamin K_2 has also been shown to improve osteoporosis. Vitamin K_1, found in green leafy vegetables, does not help prevent calcified plaque or osteoporosis, but is required for proper clotting of blood.

Kidney Stones

The presence of vitamin K in green leafy vegetables may be one reason vegetarians have a lower incidence of kidney stones.[42]

Vitamin K Deficiency

Vitamin K deficiency is associated with easy bruising and bleeding and increased risk of osteoporosis.

Antibiotics and Vitamin K

Most of your body's supply of vitamin K is synthesized by the friendly bacteria in your intestines. But when you take antibiotics, you increase your need for vitamin K. The antibiotics kill many of the good bacteria, and as a result, the remaining good bacteria cannot produce adequate amounts of vitamin K.[43]

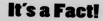

It's a Fact!

According to the USDA, only one in four Americans meet their adequate intake of vitamin K.

MAGNESIUM

MAGNESIUM IS NEEDED FOR protein, fatty acid, and bone formation, but 56 percent of Americans aren't consuming enough.[44] Magnesium is used in making new cells, in relaxing muscles, and in the clotting of blood. It helps form ATP, which gives us energy. It assists with over three hundred different enzyme reactions in the body; helps prevent muscle spasm, heart attacks, and heart disease; aids in lowering blood pressure; and eases asthma. It also helps prevent osteoporosis and helps regulate the colon and bowels. The recommended daily amount for the average person from fifteen to fifty years old is 400 mg.

Magnesium is found in nuts, seeds, dark green leafy vegetables, grains, and legumes. It is easy to see why many Americans are deficient in this important mineral, because many are eating fast foods and junk foods instead of "living foods." Common sources of magnesium include:[45]

Food	Amount of Magnesium
Halibut, 3 oz., cooked serving	90 mg
Almonds, 1 oz., dry roasted	80 mg
Cashews, 1 oz., dry roasted	75 mg
Spinach, organic, frozen, ½ cup, cooked	75 mg
Black-eyed peas, ½ cup, cooked	45 mg

Magnesium Deficiency

In order to get your reference daily intake (RDI), you would have to eat about 5 ounces of almonds every day. If you don't get enough magnesium, you may experience loss of appetite, nausea, and fatigue. If the deficiency worsens, patients may develop muscle weakness, muscle twitches, irregular heartbeat, leg cramps, insomnia, and eye twitches. Symptoms of deficiency also include constipation, headaches, personality changes, and coronary spasms, which cause chest pains. Magnesium is a building block of your health.

Bottled Water as a Source of Magnesium

Check the mineral content of your bottled water. The ideal water is water that is high in magnesium (at least 90 mg per liter) and low in sodium (less than 10 mg per liter). For example, a few waters that meet these criteria are from the same area in Northern California—Noah's California Spring Water with an incredible 120 mg of magnesium per liter, Adobe Springs water with 110 mg per liter, and BlueStar Springs, also with 110 mg magnesium per liter. For more information, go to www.mgwater.com/list5.shtml, where you will find links to these waters.

Nutrition Facts / Valeur nutritive
Per 500 mL / par 500 mL

Amount / Teneur		% Daily Value / % valeur quotidienne
Calories / Calories	0	0 %
Fat / Lipides	0 g	
Sodium / Sodium	20 mg	1 %
Carbohydrate / Glucides	0 g	0 %
Protein / Protéines	0 g	
Calcium / Calcium		4 %

Not a significant source of saturated fat, trans fat, cholesterol, fibre, sugars, vitamin A, vitamin C or iron.

Source négligeable de lipides saturés, lipides trans, cholestérol, fibres, sucres, vitamine A, vitamine C et fer.

Magnesium and Regularity

Your colon needs magnesium to help it undergo peristalsis, which propels food through and out. Most Americans don't take in adequate amounts of magnesium, fiber, and water.

CALCIUM

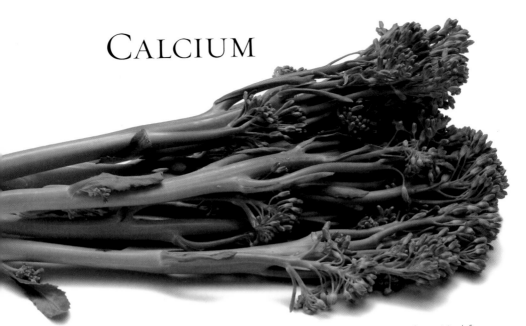

CALCIUM IS ALSO REQUIRED by your body in relatively large amounts. About 99 percent of your calcium resides in your bones and teeth. The remaining 1 percent circulates in your blood and carries out the critical function of regulating muscle contraction, heart contraction, and nerve function. Calcium gives you strong bones and prevents osteoporosis. It even lowers blood pressure. Some studies suggest that when you get adequate calcium in dietary and supplemental form, you decrease your risk of colon cancer.[46]

Children and teens age nine to eighteen need 1,300 mg a day, persons age nineteen to fifty need 1,000 mg a day, and individuals over age fifty-one need 1,200 mg a day.[47] Calcium is found in higher amounts in these foods:[48]

Food	Amount of Calcium
Yogurt, plain, low-fat, 8 oz.	415 mg
Calcium-fortified soy or rice milk, 8 oz.	80–500 mg
Turnip greens, 4 cups, boiled	396 mg
Kale, cooked, 4 cups	376 mg
Milk, nonfat, 8 fl. oz.	302 mg
Cheddar cheese, 1.5 oz.	206 mg
Tofu, firm, made with calcium sulfate, ½ cup	204 mg
Cottage cheese, 1% milkfat, 1 cup unpacked	138 mg
Spinach, ½ cup, cooked	120 mg

It's a Fact!

Studies show that more than 75 percent of Americans do not meet the current recommendations for calcium intake.[49] Low calcium intake has become a major public health problem in the United States.

Calcium Deficiency

If you don't consume enough dietary calcium, your body will eventually cannibalize the calcium from the bones to maintain calcium levels in the blood. This can quietly lead to osteopenia and osteoporosis, which literally means "porous bones"—or bones lacking in minerals and mass.

Very few women get all the calcium they need from diet, and in old age their skeletons shrink. The first bones to go are the jawbone and the vertebra in the back, which is why older people lose their teeth and height. Calcium deficiencies can also result in leg cramps, muscle cramps, and easy bruising and bleeding (since calcium is essential to blood clotting).

For more dairy recommendations, go to pages 104–105.

POTASSIUM

POTASSIUM IS A MINERAL that helps muscles contract, maintains fluid balance, sends nerve impulses, and releases energy from food. Potassium is needed to regulate blood pressure, neuromuscular function, and levels of acidity. Your body needs sodium and potassium to maintain good health. They both help regulate fluids in and out of your body cells.

According to a new report, most adults consume excessive amounts of sodium, and many don't consume enough potassium. The reason is that processed and fast foods are high in sodium, and fruits and most vegetables are high in potassium. The average American diet is lacking in fruits and vegetables. The Institute of Medicine of the National Academies of Science recently issued recommendations for sodium and potassium intake levels, saying healthy adults between

Potassium Deficiency

Eating too much salt may lower your body's store of potassium. Low potassium intake is associated with high blood pressure, irregular heartbeat, wheezing and asthma, weakness, nausea, loss of appetite, altered mental states (including nervousness and depression), dry skin, insomnia, and fatigue.

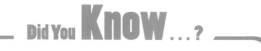

Did You Know ... ?

Less than 5 percent of the population eat more than their adequate intake of potassium.[50]

nineteen and fifty should consume about 1,500 mg of sodium per day and 4,700 mg of potassium.

Potassium is one of the main electrolytes in the body, along with sodium and chloride. These three electrolytes play a key chemical role in every function of the body. The RDI (reference daily intake) of potassium for anyone ten years old and above is 2,000 mg.[51] This means the average adult would have to eat the equivalent of three baked sweet potatoes every day to get the RDI.

Reach your recommended daily intake of potassium by adding these foods to your daily menu: fish, potatoes, avocadoes, dried apricots, bananas, citrus juices, dairy products, and whole grains. All are wonderful sources of potassium. The top foods are:[52]

Food	Amount of Potassium
Sweet potato, baked	694 mg
Tomato paste, ¼ cup	664 mg
Beet greens, ½ cup, cooked	655 mg
Yogurt, plain, nonfat, 8 oz.	579 mg
Prune juice, ¾ cup	530 mg
Carrot juice, ¾ cup	517 mg
Halibut, 3 oz., cooked	490 mg
Soybeans, green, ½ cup, cooked	485 mg
Banana, medium	422 mg
Peaches, dried, ¼ cup	398 mg
Milk, nonfat, 1 cup	382 mg
Cantaloupe, ¼ medium	368 mg
Kidney beans, ½ cup, cooked	358 mg
Orange juice, ¾ cup	355 mg

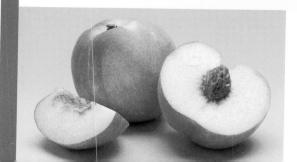

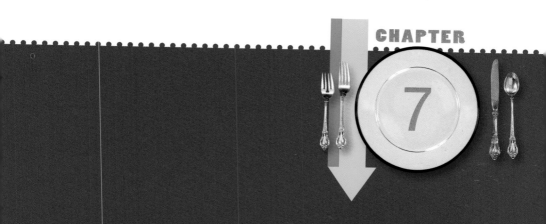

WHAT TO EAT WITH CAUTION

Why Meat Is a "Caution" Food

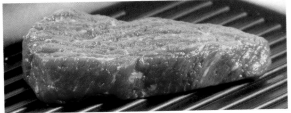

GOD CREATED US TO be omnivores, meaning we are capable of eating both plants and animals. Scientific study of the human body proves that He designed us to be better suited for consuming more plant products than animal products. Here's the evidence:

- Humans have twenty molars for grinding plant foods, eight incisors used for biting into fruits and vegetables, and only four small canine teeth designed for eating meat.

- The human intestinal tract is approximately four times longer than the average person's height, whereas a carnivore's intestinal tract is only about two to three times its body length. This longer intestinal tract in humans is evidence that we were designed to consume more plants as food.

- Our saliva is alkaline, which helps us digest carbohydrates or plant products, but a carnivore's saliva is acidic.

- A carnivore's stomach secretes as much as four times the amount of hydrochloric acid as an herbivore's stomach.

- Carnivores have larger kidneys and livers to handle excessive organic waste from animal foods. Their livers secrete more bile to break down high-fat meats.

  Nonhuman primates—monkeys, gorillas, and chimps—are omnivores, but

A Good Egg

Eggs are a great source of protein, but because cooking eggs makes the protein harder to digest, they may be associated with allergies or sensitivities. If you can "stomach" eggs, an occasional egg is good for you. Here are a few quick tips:

- Look for organic, cage-free, or omega-3 eggs. Free-range chickens are generally higher in omega-3s than corn-fed, caged chickens.

- There is no nutritional difference between brown eggs and white eggs; they are simply different colors because the hens who lay them are different colors.

- Instead of frying your eggs or scrambling them in butter or oil, try poaching or boiling them.

only rarely do they ever consume small animals, eggs, and lizards. Only about 1 percent of their total calories comes from animal foods, whereas humans consume as much as 50 percent of their calories from animal foods.

The problem is that although humans are omnivores, many of us act like carnivores. We don't understand the dangers of eating too much meat or the wrong meats. Here are the top three reasons to limit red meat in your diet.

1. Toxic fat

Red meat has a higher concentration of toxins than nearly all other foods. And any pesticide, sulfa drug, hormone, antibiotic, chemical, or other toxic residue an animal eats generally gets stored in its fat.

2. Excess protein

Eating too much protein congests your organs and cells. When you eat a 16-ounce steak or other meat, you load your body with excessive protein. Men only need 3–4 ounces of protein from meat with each meal; women need 2–3 ounces.

Excessive protein intake may put a strain on your kidneys. Therefore, individuals with kidney failure must restrict their intake of protein. Excessive protein also makes your tissues acidic, which sets the stage for arthritis, osteoporosis, and degeneration.

3. Irradiation

Irradiation is a process whereby many foods, from meats to grains to juices, are zapped with radiation equal to 10 to 70 million chest X-rays to kill or prevent microorganisms from growing.[1] The FDA has allowed poultry to be irradiated since 1990 and red meat since 1997.[2]

Irradiation destroys up to 95 percent of vitamin A in chicken, 86 percent of vitamin B in oats, and 70 percent of vitamin C in fruit juices.[3] It also reduces essential fatty acids, amino acids, friendly bacteria, and enzymes in food.[4]

Avoid foods marked with the Radura symbol— the international sign of irradiation—shown below. If no Radura symbol appears, watch for legally required warnings, such as "treated with irradiation."

Eating Out?

Here are a few restaurants that do not serve irradiated food:

- Chili's
- Macaroni Grill
- Outback Steakhouse
- Ruby Tuesday's
- Tia's Tex-Mex
- Olive Garden

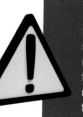

Fat Caution

For a 2,000-calorie diet, only 30 percent of your calories should come from fat.[5] Out of that 600 calories from fat, not more than 200 calories should come from saturated fat. The remaining 400 calories should come from seeds, nuts, healthy cold-pressed oils such as olive oil, and fatty fish such as wild-caught salmon.

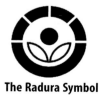

The Radura Symbol

How to Safely Eat Meat

IN SPITE OF THE dangers on the previous page, you can still enjoy meat after taking some precautions. Here are my recommendations:

> Try to choose organic, free-range, or grass-fed meat, and always look for the leanest cuts—chicken breast, turkey breast, or very lean cuts of filet mignon or tenderloin. This will help you decrease or avoid potential toxins in the fat. Free-range meats are healthiest because the animals were not fed antibiotics, growth hormones, and other toxins. The breasts of free-range chickens contain some of the lowest amounts of animal fat. Organic and free-range animals feed on grasses and have more omega-3 fats in the meat than grain-fed cattle. Grain-fed cattle are usually much fatter and contain more omega-6 fat as well as saturated fats.[6] The fat content of wild game is about 4 percent, whereas grain-fed beef typically contains 30 percent or more fat.

> If you cannot afford organic or free-range meat or poultry, get the leanest cuts, trim off any visible fat, and remove any skin. Remember, make sure the meat has not been irradiated.

> Turkey is one of the best choices of meats. Turkey breast is one of the leanest meats and contains the least amount of pesticides and toxins. Other relatively safe meats include the leanest cuts of lamb, venison (U.S.), rabbit, and buffalo.

> Some people worry about giving up meat because they wrongly believe they won't get enough protein in their diet. But a balanced diet that includes small amounts of lean meats and generous portions of beans and whole grains can give you the protein you need. For example, whole-grain bread and hummus make a complete protein when eaten together. Remember, only about 1 percent of a gorilla's diet is derived from animal meat.

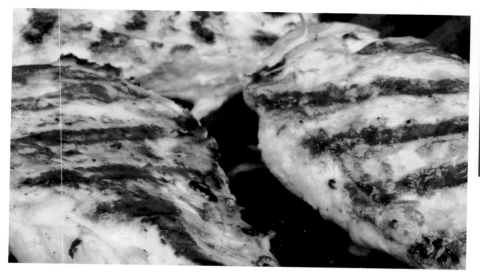

> If you choose to eat red meats, limit them to only 4 to 6 ounces, once or twice a week. A diet high in red meat is associated with an increased risk of breast[7] and prostate[8] cancers.

> When preparing poultry, trim off the skin and any visible fat before it is cooked. If you leave the fat and skin on, the pesticides collected in these parts of the animal may seep into the meat. Bake, broil, grill, or lightly stir-fry your meat. (Don't deep-fry your chickens or turkeys, as some people have begun doing.) Scrape off charred portions, because char contains benzopyrenes, which are carcinogens and are associated with colorectal cancer.

> Cook meats thoroughly since most poultry contains dangerous bacteria such as salmonella, campylobacteria, and staphylococcus, which are associated with food poisoning.

Once you start buying the right kinds of meats and preparing them in a healthy way, you can fully enjoy them as part of your regular diet.

Dr. Colbert Approved

Red Meats
- Lean cuts only
- Organically raised preferred
- Hormone free
- Scrape off the char if you grill it

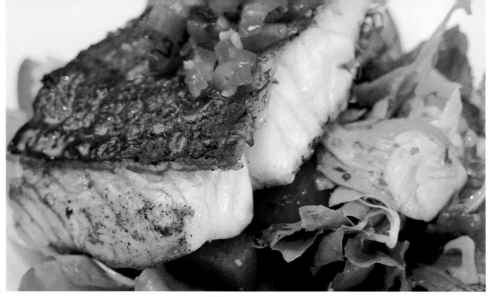

FISH

I USED TO RECOMMEND fish much more heartily than I do now, but new studies keep emerging about the high mercury content of fish, even fish formerly considered safe. For that reason I'm much more cautious now about fish.

Because the oceans, lakes, and rivers have suffered from the toxic onslaught of chemicals along with the rest of the environment, fish are no longer free of toxins. The American College of Obstetricians and Gynecologists recommends only two 6-ounce servings of fish a week for pregnant women,[9] and the American Academy of Pediatrics recommends no more than 7 ounces of fish a week.[10] This is because fish increasingly contains mercury, which is toxic for the fetus and for children's brains.

But if you are careful about which fish you eat,

Dr. Colbert Approved

Fish

Here is a list of some fish that are usually pesticide free:

- Wild Alaskan or Pacific salmon
- Mahimahi (Florida)
- Sardines
- Rainbow trout (farm raised)
- Tongol tuna
- Grouper (Argentina, Chile, Mexico)

they can be your best source of healthy omega-3 oils, which study after study has shown is one of the best oils on the planet. Here are my recommendations:

- Fish with the highest concentrations of omega-3 oils are Pacific herring, king salmon, wild Pacific salmon, anchovies, and lake trout. Wild Pacific salmon contains higher omega-3 fat than farm-raised Atlantic salmon.

- Look into buying tongol tuna, which is much lower in mercury and comes from much smaller tuna. Most store-bought tuna comes from larger tunas, which contain much higher mercury content. Tongol tuna is generally found in health food stores.

- Other good fish are tilapia, halibut, grouper, striped sea bass, and sole.

- Avoid shark and sword-fish. They have some of the highest levels of mercury and pesti-cides of any fish in the sea. Sharks will eat anything, and they eat a lot of pesticides. In many areas trout have also been subjected to contamination through industrialization. Use caution, and select fish taken from fresh, pure-water areas.

Tips for Selecting Fish

If you purchase your fish from a grocery store, use wisdom. Nearly 40 percent of your grocer's fish may have already begun to spoil. Ensure the quality of your purchases by using this brief checklist:

- Look for shiny, bright, bulging fish. If the scales are shiny, the fish is typically good.

- The flesh should spring back. If your thumb leaves an indentation, don't buy it.

- If it smells fishy, don't buy it.

- If the fish has not been kept on ice at 32 degrees, don't buy it.

- Certain ocean waters are known for their purity. The waters of Australia are extremely pure, as are the waters of Chile. The seas surrounding New Zealand and Greece are also extremely clean. Most fish you purchase from these waters should be safe to eat.

- Shrimp contains higher levels of cholesterol than other seafood, but it is usually free from contamination from pesticides, though it usually contains the heavy metal cadmium, which is associated with hypertension. Most shellfish contain cadmium, so if you choose to eat shellfish, do so infrequently and eat those from less-industrialized areas where the waters remain uncontaminated.

DAIRY PRODUCTS

MANY PEOPLE EAT DAIRY products with great abandon because they associate milk with health, robustness, and wholesomeness. But from a physician's point of view, I'm highly aware of the problems caused by dairy products. Most children I see in my practice with chronic ear infections and sinus infections have dairy sensitivities. Other doctors I know of say that eliminating dairy products is often the only thing they need to do to stop recurrent ear problems in children. One doctor reported that, of all the children he saw who required tubes to be put into their eardrums for drainage purposes, three out of four did not need the tubes when they stopped eating dairy products.[11]

Dairy products, and cow's milk in particular, are also linked to allergies and sensitivities, including skin rashes, eczema, fatigue, spastic colon, excessive mucus production, nasal allergies, and chronic sinus infections. Some people even have diarrhea due to lactose intolerance. If you (or especially children) have any of these, stop all dairy products—including skim milk, butter, and even yogurt—for a week or so, and watch the improvement. Small wonder

You'll find more tips about dairy on pages 126–127.

that man is the only species in the animal kingdom to drink cow's milk as an adult.

Another problem with milk is that it is pasteurized by heating it at 161 degrees for fifteen seconds, which denatures milk enzymes and changes its protein structure, making it difficult for our bodies to assimilate and digest.[12] However, I do not recommend raw milk since it may contain toxic bacteria such as *Brucella*, which is associated with brucellosis.[13]

Finally, dairy products tend to have lots of saturated fat, which is associated with high cholesterol and heart disease. Butter is 81 percent saturated fat. Cheese is 75 percent fat. Regular milk is 4 percent saturated fat, which means that 48 percent of its calories come from fat—way too high for a healthy diet.

Should dairy products be banished

from your diet? Not necessarily. Here are tips to eating healthy dairy products.

- Consider goat's milk. Goat's milk products generally cause fewer allergies and sensitivities than cow's milk. Even though it is difficult to obtain organic, low-fat, or fat-free goat's milk or goat cheese, it can be found in some health food stores and online. Grocery stores will often order a product for customers who request it, so don't be afraid to inquire at your local store.

- Choose organic skim dairy products. They have no saturated fat, and they are much lower in calories. Eat low-fat or nonfat organic dairy products like cheese, sour cream, yogurt, kefir, and so on. Use small amounts of organic butter or ghee, which is clarified butter. It's best to avoid ice cream and frozen yogurt since they are generally high in sugar, and ice cream is usually high in sugar and saturated fat.

Lactose Intolerant?

Some people can't digest dairy products, so here are some other foods high in calcium:

Sardines, canned, ½ cup (3½ oz.)	314 mg
Red salmon, ½ cup (3½ oz.)	259 mg
Pink salmon, ½ cup (3½ oz.)	196 mg
Mustard greens, cooked (½ cup)	138 mg
Broccoli, cooked (1 large stalk)	88 mg
Collard greens, cooked (½ cup)	152 mg
Turnip greens, cooked (½ cup)	138 mg
Spinach, cooked (½ cup)	107 mg
Bok choy (½ cup)	126 mg

- Eat kefir and yogurt from time to time if you are not sensitive to dairy. I believe the best dairy product for you is low-fat organic kefir or yogurt, which contain good bacteria that help maintain a healthy GI tract. Eat a small container of yogurt a few times a week, but not the high-sugar, high-fat variety. Most packaged yogurt is just dessert in a yogurt cup. Instead, buy plain low-fat organic yogurt or goat's milk organic yogurt and add your own fresh fruit.

Most mornings, as part of my breakfast I blend one organic apple with 6 ounces of low-fat, plain, organic kefir and 1 to 2 tablespoons of ground flaxseeds. This makes a tasty smoothie with ten strains of beneficial bacteria and lots of fiber.

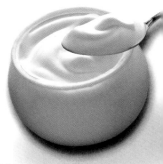

IS CAFFEINE BAD?

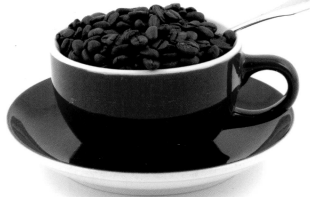

COFFEE, COLA, AND TEA are not substitutes for water, but recent studies also show that caffeine isn't all bad for you. It helps prevent Parkinson's disease and cirrhosis of the liver, and it helps with male fertility. It has also been shown to protect the brain, possibly from diseases like Alzheimer's.[14] A Harvard study showed that the risk for developing type 2 diabetes is lower among regular coffee drinkers.[15] Coffee also is linked to lower rates of suicide, colon cancer, high blood pressure in women, and heart disease.[16] People who drink decaffeinated coffee also show reduced diabetes risk, though at half the benefit of those drinking caffeinated coffee.[17]

The key, as with anything, is moderation. One or two cups a day won't hurt you, but three to four cups may be too much. You can drink coffee or iced tea all day and still be mildly dehydrated, because caffeine is a diuretic, meaning it removes water from the body. Some individuals with arrhythmias of the heart, fibrocystic breast disease, and migraine headaches should probably avoid caffeinated beverages altogether.[18]

If you don't like coffee—and even if you do—you should drink organic green tea or white tea. Green tea has been a favorite in Japan for over a thousand years. Its antioxidant activity is two hundred times more potent than that of vitamin E and five hundred times more potent than vitamin C. This decreases the risk of cancer. Have two or three cups of organic green tea a day.

The newest tea sensation is white tea. Like all teas, white tea is harvested from the *Camellia sinensis* plant, but white tea is harvested before the fresh white buds of the tea plant have matured. While black tea is fully fermented and green tea is only partly fermented, white tea is not fermented at all. Therefore, it offers even more cancer-fighting antioxidants than green tea. Some studies show that it contains up to three times as much antioxidant power as green tea and twelve times as much as fresh orange juice.[19]

Dr. Colbert Approved

Coffee

Here's a recipe for healthy coffee. Use unbleached (brown) filters, organic coffee, alkaline water, and stevia instead of sugar. If you must have a creamer, use organic skim milk or rice milk, and never use a Styrofoam cup, as styrene, considered a possible human carcinogen, tends to migrate into food and beverages more quickly if they are hot.[20] Also, I recommend Farberware's coffee maker, which is stainless steel, instead of the typical plastic auto-drip coffee makers.

NOTE: Avoid specialty coffee drinks. These drinks are loaded with calories, fat, and sugar. A small muffin and a mocha frap from some coffee shops can supply amost a whole day's worth of calories!

Organic Is Best

Most teas contain pesticides as well as fluorides. The pesticides in the tea may be canceling out the powerful antioxidant effects of the tea. Wine is usually loaded with pesticides, and so is nonorganic coffee. If you choose to drink tea, wine, and coffee, then I recommend drinking only organic teas, wines, and coffees in moderation. To make sure you can always choose organic tea wherever you go, simply carry some organic tea bags in your purse.

Good News, Chocoholics!

The *British Medical Journal* reported in 1998 that dark chocolate consumption is linked to longer life. It has been shown to reduce blood pressure and bad cholesterol. It opens blood vessels and allows blood to circulate more freely, which is good for heart health.[21]

Cacao beans are high in antioxidants. Chocolate has more antioxidants than fruits, vegetables, tea, and wine. One study showed that people who ate 3 ounces of dark chocolate every day for three weeks had lower blood pressure and improved insulin sensitivity.[22]

Provided you do not have a weight problem, eating 1 to 3 ounces per day is good for you! Eat only chocolate that has:

- 60 percent or higher cocoa content
- Low sugar levels
- All organic ingredients
- No dairy content

WHAT TO DRINK

WATER: THE MIRACLE CURE

WATER IS THE SINGLE most important nutrient for our bodies. It is involved in every function of our bodies. You can live five to seven weeks without food, but the average adult can last no more than five days without water.[1]

Many people never drink water. Some don't like the taste of water, or they were never taught the impor-tance of drinking it. They live in a mildly dehydrated state with various irritating symptoms and never realize it. I often tell patients that when they have a headache, they don't have a Tylenol deficiency. When they have joint pain, they don't have an Advil deficiency. When they have heartburn, they don't have a Pepcid deficiency, and if they are depressed, they don't have a Prozac deficiency. In each of these cases, their body is often crying out for water.[2]

I treat every patient I see in my practice first with water. Most of my patients get better when they simply drink the water their body is asking for. Drinking sufficient amounts of the right kind of water will also do more to improve your health than anything else you can do.

H_2O 101
Your body loses about two quarts of water a day through perspiration, urination, and exhalation.[3]

Did You **Know**...?

- Your body is about 70 percent water.

- Your muscles are about 75 percent water.

- Your brain cells are about 85 percent water.

- Your blood is approximately 82 percent water.

- Even your bones are approximately 25 percent water.[4]

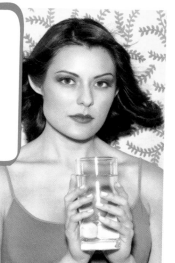

It's a Fact!

Water plays a vital role in regulating body temperature, transporting nutrients and oxygen to cells, removing waste, cushioning joints, and protecting organs and tissues.[5]

Take a Guess

Which food is highest in water content?

a. Watermelon

b. Lettuce

c. Grapefruit

Answer: b. Lettuce. Although all of the foods listed have a high percentage of water content, a half-cup of lettuce has the highest at 95 percent.[6]

Wet Behind the Ears?

What percentage of water does the average adult male body contain?

a. 50–55 percent

b. 55–62 percent

c. 62–65 percent

Answer: c. The average adult male's body is 62–65 percent water, compared to women, who have 51–55 percent water. Men have more water in their bodies because they generally have more muscle mass, whereas women have a higher percentage of body fat.

WATER: HOW MUCH AND HOW OFTEN?

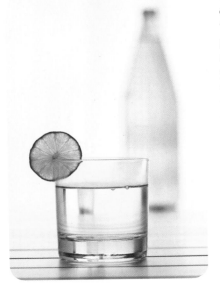

OUR BODIES YEARN FOR pure, clean water. But one of the most common questions I hear is, "How much water should I drink?" I'm going to give you the answer to that question. To determine how much water your body needs, take your body weight (in pounds) and divide it by two. That's how many ounces of water you need every day—unless you have congestive heart failure or kidney failure, in which case you should consult your physician.

Usually, that amounts to two or three quarts a day. Picture a one-gallon container of milk, and imagine it three-quarters full. If you are an average-sized person, that's about how much water your body needs daily. If you weigh 120 pounds, you will need 60 ounces of water; if 220 pounds, you'll need 110 ounces. Most people have no idea they require that much.

But you won't consume it all in liquid form. Simply by eating lots of fruits and vegetables—as you should—you will typically get a quart a day. Foods such as bananas are 70 percent water; apples, 80 percent water; tomatoes and watermelons are more than 90 percent water; and lettuce is 95 percent water. If you eat an inordinate amount of starches, like breads or pastries, you will need more water, because these foods add little water to your body.

When to drink water

Most people wait until they are thirsty or until they have a dry mouth before they take a drink. By that time you are most likely already mildly dehydrated. A dry mouth is one of the last signs of dehydration.

Other people only drink during meals—another mistake. When you drink too much with a meal, it washes out the hydrochloric acid, digestive juices, and enzymes in your

How Much Should I Drink?

Take your weight in pounds and divide it by two. The result is how many ounces of water you should drink daily.

_____ Weight ÷ 2 = _____ ounces per day

stomach and intestines, which delays digestion. Fluids, and iced drinks in particular, quench the digestive process similarly to pouring water on a fire.

You can drink some water with a meal. I usually drink room-temperature unsweetened tea or bottled water with a slice of lemon or lime squeezed into it. But don't go overboard. Meals are not the time to get most of your fluids. Stick to 4 to 8 ounces with a meal.

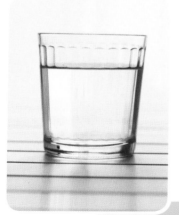

Best Times to Drink Water

Here's a typical timetable for healthy water consumption:

- Start with 8 to 16 ounces half an hour before breakfast. If you usually have juice, coffee, or tea with breakfast, don't eliminate them. The point is not to take the fun out of life. You don't want to feel like a slave to water, but do limit coffee to one or two cups a day if you can. Organic green tea, white tea, or black tea only have a small amount of caffeine, 30 and 50 mg per 8-ounce serving. So you can have a few glasses of tea a day, though not late in the evening, as it may interfere with your sleep, or you may choose decaf organic teas.

- A couple of hours after breakfast, drink another 8 to 16 ounces of water.

- Then thirty minutes before your evening meal drink your next glass. If dinner is your largest meal of the day, try drinking 16 to 24 ounces (or if lunch is your big meal, drink 16 to 24 ounces before that meal). I predict that you won't eat as much.

- Finally, two hours after dinner, have another 8 ounces and another before bedtime, unless you have a hiatal hernia, reflux disease, an enlarged prostate, or frequent urination during the night. In those cases, do not drink anything else after dinner.

Climate Matters

If you live in a warmer or drier climate, you will need more water. Most of us lose about a pint of water a day through perspiration. Our bodies also lose water through exhalation (about a pint a day) and through urination and stool (about one to two pints a day).[8] Two pints equal one quart, so our bodies lose about one and a half to two quarts a day. However, this doesn't account for excessive perspiration.

BOTTLED WATER

MANY PEOPLE DRINK BOTTLED water instead of tap water, making bottled water the second most popular beverage in the United States behind soft drinks.[9] People today consume twice as much bottled water as they did a decade ago, and the growth in the bottled water industry is "unparalleled," according to the Beverage Marketing Corporation.[10]

But is bottled water healthier for you? Does that attractive bottle with the pictures of snowy mountains and crystal-line streams really mean the water inside is pure?

Less Regulated Than Tap

Bottled water is considered a food; there-fore, it is regulated by the FDA. Tap water is regulated by the EPA.[11] The only requirement placed on bottled water is that it be as safe as tap water. But while the EPA makes cities test public drinking water daily, the FDA requires only yearly testing for bottled water.[12] The EPA forbids the presence of bacteria, which indicate the presence of fecal material, but the FDA has no such rule, meaning bottled water can contain fecal bacteria and still be legal.[13]

More Toxins Than Tap

A study of one hundred brands of bottled water showed that a third contained arsenic, trihalomethanes, bacteria, or other contaminants. A fifth contained man-made chemicals, and one contained phthalate at twice the level acceptable in tap water. Two had high levels of fluoride, and two others had coliform bacteria.[14] And if you think that bottled water is lead free, think again. The FDA allows bottled water to contain up to five parts per billion of lead.[15]

More Information About Bottled Water

If you are going to drink bottled water, make sure the bottler is a member of the International Bottled Water Association (IBWA), which guarantees that the level of contaminants, if any, is below FDA standards. Go to the IBWA Web site at www.bottledwater.org to see which bottled water makers are members.

Some helpful Web sites that compare many different bottled waters are:

- www.tldp.com/issue/190/Bottled%20Water.htm
- www.AquaMaestro.com
- www.mineralwaters.org

Dr. Colbert Approved

Penta Water

Penta Water, found in health food stores, is considered the purest bottled water on the market. I find it especially beneficial for my patients with fibromyalgia, chronic fatigue, headaches, arthritis, and most degenerative diseases. I usually recommend 16 ounces of Penta Water a day, along with one to two quarts of pure spring water.

Glass or Bioplastic Bottles

Because studies continue to show that that some forms of plastic are not as safe as people believe, I prefer drinking water from glass bottles or from bio-based plastics, which are made from natural products. In 2005, one bottled water company, Biota, introduced the use of the first compostable bioplastic bottle. I suspect that many other companies will follow suit.

I discuss the safety of various types of plastics in greater detail in my book *The Seven Pillars of Health*. The topic and debate over which plastics are safest will continue, and so will the recommendations. As for now, the safest plastics to use are PET (or PETE) and bioplastics.

Where Bottled Water Really Comes From

Dasani and Aquafina waters, two of the biggest brands in America, are reprocessed tap water from cities around the country. One of Aquafina's sources is the Detroit River![16] About one-fourth of bottled water is tap water, according to government and industry estimates.[17]

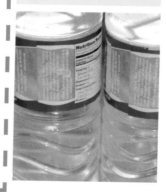

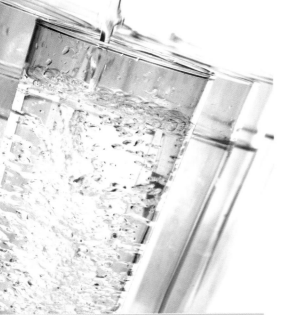

Filtered Water

ONE OF THE BEST kinds of water to drink is filtered water. Using a water filter in your home can be a big step toward restoring health to your drinking water. Some people use filtration pitchers or faucet-mounted carbon filters, some use full-home filtration systems, and others use reverse-osmosis under-the-counter systems and distillation. These may sound mysterious and expensive, but a good water filter probably costs less than you currently spend on soft drinks every month. However, not all filtration systems are created equal. On these two pages, I rank what I think are the healthiest kinds of water filtration options from one star (OK) to five stars (my top recommendation).

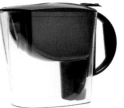

Carbon Filters ★

Carbon filters come in many forms, from a water-filtering pitcher to a faucet-mounted filter, and are the "entry-level" filters: inexpensive, but incomplete, in my opinion.

If you choose a carbon filter, you remove most chlorine and 90 percent of lead from your tap water, but many toxins—fluoride, viruses, pharmaceuticals, personal care products—are not filtered out.[18] Also, if you don't change the filters as the instructions direct, they can become more of a hazard than a help, by collecting the "garbage" in the water and breeding bacteria.[19]

Water Distillers ★ ★

Water distillers are extremely effective at removing everything—unfortunately even good minerals—from water.[20] The water is mineral free. A growing body of evidence suggests that completely mineral-free water is worse for your body than water with dissolved minerals in it.

A distiller will get you halfway to your goal. You won't have anything bad in your water, but it can adversely affect your health in other ways.

Reverse Osmosis ★★★

In terms of price, reverse-osmosis systems are the "optimum level" of water filters. They filter water through an extremely fine membrane, and like distillers, they remove virtually everything from water. The acidic water they produce is similar to distilled water. It is 95 percent mineral free, acidic, and therefore aggressive—meaning it pulls minerals from anything with which it comes in contact. Because the water is acidic, it may keep your tissues acidic.[21]

Both distilled water and reverse-osmosis water are the purest water. If you use these filtering methods, make sure that you take adequate minerals. It's also a good idea to add an alkaline booster to your water. A couple of drops in an 8-ounce glass of water will raise the alkalinity to a healthy level. You can purchase these drops from most health food stores.

Dr. Colbert Approved

Variety of Filters
★★★★★

I use a variety of filters and spring waters because each has its unique benefits. I always start with spring water that is alkaline because it supplies minerals in their natural form. For everyday drinking I use Mountain Valley Spring brand bottled water. When I go to the gym, I take a bottle of Penta Water with me. When I make coffee, I use an alkalizing filter, because coffee is acidic. At home I use reverse-osmosis water in my ice machine. I also have a filter outside of the house for all water entering the house because simply taking a shower with tap water causes you to inhale chlorine, which may be roughly equivalent to drinking a gallon of chlorinated tap water. If a whole-house filtration system is not in your budget, then please at least consider purchasing a shower filter.

Alkaline Water Filters ★★★★

Your body thrives in an alkaline environment since your tissues get rid of impurities more efficiently. I use an alkalizing filter in my home and office. Because a water alkalizer uses an electromagnetic process to separate acidic water from alkaline water, the water you put into it must be rich in minerals and not distilled or reverse-osmosis water.

Some alkalizer filters also make the water clustered or "hexagonal," meaning that at a molecular level, it is denser, richer, and more energetic. All of these attributes benefit health in many ways. For more information on this topic, refer to my book *The Seven Pillars of Health.* I have recommended alkaline, hexagonal water to my patients for years.

Certain bottled waters are also alkaline. Evamor and Abita waters are just a few of the alkaline bottled waters.

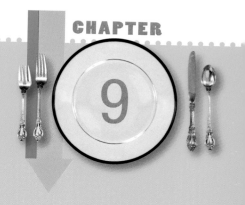

SHOPPING TIPS

PLANNING AHEAD

IT DOES TAKE MORE EFFORT to eat healthily; however, you can reduce the amount of time you spend preparing healthy meals with a little preparation and planning. Follow these steps: (1) purge your fridge, pantry, and kitchen cabinets of all unhealthy, dead, processed foods; (2) read labels to watch for hidden sources of sugar and additives like MSG; (3) keep a shopping list at the ready, and as you run out of items throughout the week, add them to the list; (4) to move your family toward healthier eating, plan to serve at least one meatless meal during the week and include one dessert that consists primarily of fruit; and (5) stock healthy staples in your kitchen so that last-minute meals don't have to be made from dead foods. Add these staple items to your shopping list if they are missing or running low:

Pantry

- Extra-virgin olive oil and other cold-pressed healthy oils (choose organic when available)
- Organic dried or canned beans of many varieties (when selecting canned versions, stay away from any that have added animal fat, salt, or other preservatives)
- Whole-grain, high-fiber pastas, sandwich breads, cereals, and crackers
- Salt-free natural seasonings (remember to look for nonirradiated products)
- Organic coffee and tea
- Organic nuts and seeds
- Organic garlic, onions, and potatoes

Fridge

- Frozen veggies (avoid canned as much as possible)
- Low-fat dairy options (skim milk, low-fat cheese, plain kefir and yogurt, etc.)
- Fresh, organic fruits and vegetables (don't buy too much; it's better to make frequent trips to the store every couple of days so you are eating fresh produce, not produce that has been sitting in your fridge for five days)
- Lean, organic, free-range meats and wild-caught fish

Nonfood items

- Juicer (look for one that allows you to add pulp back into the juice after juicing)
- Mister (great way to spray olive oil on veggies before roasting or grilling and for spraying healthy dressing on your salad)
- Pitcher-style water filter (if you can't invest in a whole-house filtration system off the bat, this is an economical way to start filtering your water)

Before You Shop

- Before going to the grocery store, always eat a healthy, well-balanced meal or snack containing plenty of fiber so that your stomach is full. Nothing will tempt you to load up on unhealthy foods more than shopping on an empty stomach!

- Don't forget your shopping list! This will make it more likely that you will stay away from impulse buys that tend to be unhealthy.

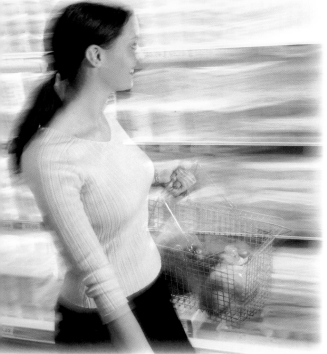

AT THE STORE

WHEN YOU'RE IN THE store, stick to your prepared grocery list and follow these tips:

✓ Stay away from the inner aisles that are loaded with boxes of processed, man-made food products. The living foods are all around the perimeter of the store! This should be where you spend the majority of your time shopping.

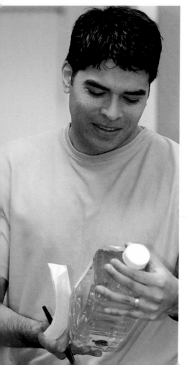

✓ If you do have to venture into the inner aisles to look for a healthy cereal option or some other whole-grain food, remember that most living food items are found high and low on the shelves, whereas dead, processed convenience foods take up the most prominent spots in the middle shelves.

✓ Frozen fruits and vegetables are an acceptable option. Be cautious if choosing frozen dinners, and read the nutrition labels carefully. You'll see my recommendations for some acceptable frozen meal options in a few pages.

✓ Read labels! Read labels! Read labels! Use the label decoder on the facing page to help you make the wisest choices.

✓ Beware of the tempting aroma of the bakery section with its doughnuts, pastries, cakes, and pies.

Nutrition Labels Decoded

You can make better food choices at the store when you understand what all the information on the Nutrition Facts panel means. Here's a quick decoder:

- TOTAL CARBOHYDRATE on a food label includes fiber and sugars, whether they occur naturally in the food or have been added.

- DIETARY FIBER is something most Americans need to increase in their diets. This score on the nutrition label tells you how much nondigestible carbohydrates are in your food.

- TOTAL FAT/SATURATED FAT/TRANS FAT/CHOLESTEROL are nutrients that are associated with chronic illness such as cancer, heart disease, and high blood pressure. Use the nutrition label to choose foods that are low in these nutrients. Be especially wary of trans fats.

- SUGAR includes naturally occurring sugars and added sugars. If you are concerned about added sugars, instead of the nutrition label, watch for added sugars listed within the first three ingredients. (Don't forget to look for other names for sugar like corn syrup, high-fructose corn syrup, fruit juice concentrate, maltose, dextrose, sucrose, honey, and maple syrup.)

- SALT is also called sodium, sodium chloride, sodium caseinate, monosodium glutamate, trisodium phosphate, sodium ascorbate, sodium bicarbonate, and sodium stearoyl lactylate. For a product to be "sodium free," it must contain less than 5 mg of sodium per serving; "very low sodium" contains 35 mg or less per serving; "low sodium" products contain 140 mg or less per serving.

- CALORIES/CALORIES FROM FAT tells you how much energy you get from a serving and helps you control your calorie intake. The "calories" category shows the total caloric content, including calories from fat, protein, and carbs. The "calories from fat" category breaks out how many of those calories are specifically from fat. A general rule of thumb is that a total calorie count of 40 calories or less is considered "low calorie"; 400 calories or more is "high calorie."

- SERVING SIZE refers to a set amount that the FDA recognizes as being commonly consumed for a particular food. It's important to remember that the nutrition information on the label is given according to serving size, not container size.

- PERCENT DAILY VALUE (% DV) tells you how much a serving contributes toward 100 percent of the daily amount you should consume for each nutrient.

Start With Produce, Meats, and Fish

PURCHASE FRUITS AND VEGETABLES frequently rather than storing large quantities for days and days in your refrigerator. And don't fall into the trap of buying the same fruits and vegetables each week. Try something different. Choose a variety of colors of fruits and vegetables, since each color offers unique protective phytonutrients and antioxidants.

Purchase fresh herbs like organic cilantro, parsley, and basil instead of using the dried varieties. Consider growing your own herbs in a planter box at home. Visit your local nursery for advice on how best to grow fresh herbs.

Don't be overly concerned about the glycemic zone values of fruits and vegetables. With the exception of potatoes and a few fruits like papaya, pineapple, and watermelon, most fruits and vegetables are low-glycemic. (And you can still eat papayas, pineapples, and watermelons even though they are not low-glycemic.)

Think Outside the Grocery Store

Most of the food we purchase in the grocery store has traveled more than 1,500 miles from the farm where it was grown.[1] Almost every grocery store receives 85 to 90 percent of its food from outside its state lines. Farmer's markets are an option to consider. They bypass the long-distance shipping and are located all over the country. They often offer as much—if not more—variety as the grocery store chains.

Another great source of fresh fruits and vegetables is community-supported agriculture (CSA), where you buy directly from local farmers who sell organic produce. For more information about CSAs or to locate one near you, visit www.nal.usda.gov/afsic/pubs/csa/csa.shtml.

Meats, poultry, and seafood

The most important thing in choosing meat is to choose the leanest cuts. As I explained earlier, I prefer organic, free-range meat and poultry. Choose free-range or organic lean ground beef, fillets, tenderloins, and roasts. Be sure to ask your butcher to trim off all visible fat. You can also purchase lean roast beef at the deli.

Choose nitrite- and nitrate-free luncheon meats. Chicken and turkey are good choices. Nitrite- and nitrate-free chicken strips are also available to make fajitas or to stir-fry.

As for seafood, choose wild fish instead of farm-raised. I recommend small tuna or tongol tuna, found in many health food stores, because it is generally very low in mercury content. Shellfish (shrimp, crab, lobsters, oyster, etc.) may be eaten on occasion, but make sure that it is cooked well.

If you are careful to select the leanest cuts of pork and ask your butcher to trim off all visible fat, it's

Go Skinless

Removing the skin from your chicken can cut your calorie and fat intake in half. But did you ever wonder whether you should remove it before or after cooking? It doesn't affect the calorie or fat content by much if you cook the chicken with the skin on, so you may want to wait to remove the skin after cooking—especially if you're cooking chicken parts that tend to dry out, such as the breast. Cooking with the skin intact keeps the meat more moist and tender.

OK to eat ham, lean pork chops, pork roast, and pork tenderloin from time to time. Avoid sausage and bacon because they are high in saturated fat. But certain nitrite-free turkey bacon, such as Apple-gate Farms organic turkey bacon, is acceptable and absolutely delicious. You may also eat Cornish hens, veal, lamb, duck, bison, or elk—all meats that are typically low in fat.

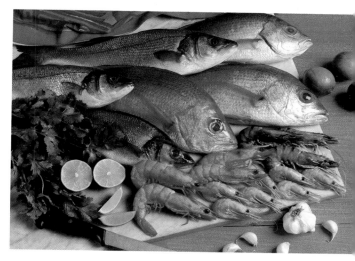

DAIRY DOS AND DON'TS

WITH THE EXCEPTION OF those who are allergic or sensitive to dairy or who are lactose intolerant, most people enjoy dairy. There are, however, both healthy and unhealthy choices you can make in selecting dairy. Here are my recommendations.

If you are able to, always opt for organic dairy foods. If these items are too expensive, however, you can choose regular fat-free or low-fat dairy.

For organic, low-fat or fat-free milk, try a brand such as Horizon Organic. They offer low-fat, fat-free, and lactose-free milk, as well as a wide variety of organic dairy products.

You should opt for fat-free cottage cheese, ricotta cheese, and part-skim milk cheese as well. For cheese that is only 35 calories per serving, check out the line of light cheese wedges from Laughing Cow.

I strongly recommend low-fat or fat-free plain kefir or yogurt. Flavored yogurts and yogurts with fruit have the sugar equivalent of a candy bar; buy plain, nonfat yogurt instead. Mix with fresh fruit, cinnamon, agave nectar, or other natural ingredients to add flavor at home.

In addition, choose organic butter over the regular kind, but use it sparingly since it is high in fat.

If Dairy Makes You Congested

As I mentioned on page 104, studies have linked dairy products with recurring ear infections in some children.[3] The ear infections are the result of congestion that occurs when dairy products cause swelling that blocks the nasal passages. I've found that some patients are able to put an end to recurring ear infections in their children simply by removing dairy from their diet.

Whether you experience ear infections or not, if drinking or eating dairy products gives you congestion, you may find relief if you:

- Eliminate all cheese products—especially pizza—for a period of three months, since cheese tends to be the main culprit that triggers the congestion.

- If congestion persists after eliminating cheese from your diet, try eliminating all dairy for the same time period and use only organic products when you reintroduce dairy to your diet.

- If symptoms persist after reintroducing dairy, as a final resort, switch to organic skim cow's milk or switch to goat's milk and goat's cheese.

- Surprisingly, some of my patients never experience relief. If none of the above steps relieve your congestion, you may need to stay away from dairy and substitute rice milk, almond milk, or small amounts of soy milk or soy cheese in place of dairy.

Antibiotics and Livestock

According to the Union of Concerned Scientists, 70 percent of the 35 million pounds of antibiotics administered each year in this country is used to stimulate growth and prevent disease in healthy livestock. The American Medical Association has opposed the use of antibiotics in agriculture on healthy animals.[2]

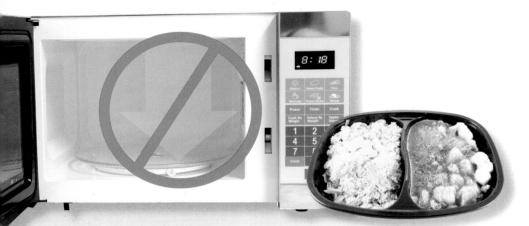

THE FREEZER AISLE: AN ACCEPTABLE OPTION

WHILE FRESH FOOD IS still the best choice for living foods, frozen foods are an acceptable second choice because freezing preserves more nutrients than allowing fresh foods to become overripe, or processing them into canned or jarred products. One of the most important factors in finding a good frozen product is learning how to read the Nutrition Facts label to make sure the item is healthy. Selecting frozen fruits and vegetables is a pretty straightforward process—you look at a bag of frozen peas, and if the ingredients list says "Peas," you're good to go! But finding healthy frozen dinner entrees is a little more complex.

There are some acceptable frozen meal options, which I've chosen because of their scores in the calorie, sodium, fat, protein, and fiber content departments. I've tried to keep these as healthy as possible, but it is very difficult, if not impossible, to find a frozen dinner that is 100 percent healthy. After all, frozen dinners should not be our staple diet, but used on occasion for convenience. It's important to limit them to once or twice a week. Remember, moderation is the key.

NOTE: Please keep in mind that some packages listed in the sidebar contain more than a single serving.

Don't Nuke Your Frozen Food!

I do not recommend that you microwave frozen foods. If the package provides directions for heating in a conventional oven, follow them. If not, most of my patients report success in heating frozen entrées in a conventional, convection, or toaster oven by simply removing the frozen food from its cardboard or plastic container, placing it in an oven-safe dish, and baking it at a low temperature, such as 350 degrees Fahrenheit, for about 20–30 minutes, watching carefully to avoid burning.

FROZEN ENTREES

BIRDS EYE VOILA!

- Pasta Primavera With Chicken: 260 calories, 660 mg sodium, 7 g fat, 32 g carbs, 15 g protein, 2 g fiber

HEALTHY CHOICE CAFÉ STEAMERS

- Creamy Dill Salmon: 240 calories, 600 mg sodium, 6 g fat, 26 g carbs, 19 g protein, 5 g fiber

HEALTHY CHOICE COMPLETE SELECTIONS

- Chicken Broccoli Alfredo: 300 calories, 430 mg sodium, 5 g fat, 46 g carbs, 17 g protein, 8 g fiber
- Traditional Turkey Breast: 300 calories, 550 mg sodium, 4 g fat, 42 g carbs, 21 g protein, 6 g fiber

HEALTHY CHOICE SIMPLE SELECTIONS

- Chicken Fettuccini Alfredo: 210 calories, 570 mg sodium, 5 g fat, 23 g carbs, 16 g protein, 5 g fiber
- Sesame Chicken: 230 calories, 600 mg sodium, 4 g fat, 34 g carbs, 13 g protein, 5 g fiber

KASHI

- Black Bean Mango: 340 calories, 430 mg sodium, 8 g fat, 58 g carbs, 8 g protein, 7 g fiber

- Chicken Pasta Pomodoro: 280 calories, 470 mg sodium, 6 g fat, 38 g carbs, 19 g protein, 6 g fiber

STOUFFER'S LEAN CUISINE

- Grilled Chicken with Teriyaki Glaze: 280 calories, 650 mg sodium, 3 g fat, 45 g carbs, 17 g protein, 2 g fiber
- Alfredo Pasta With Chicken and Broccoli: 260 calories, 660 mg sodium, 6 g fat, 34 g carbs, 17 g protein, 3 g fiber
- Chicken Florentine Lasagna: 290 calories, 650 mg sodium, 6 g fat, 37 g carbs, 21 g protein, 3 g fiber

WEIGHT WATCHERS SMART ONES

- Chicken Parmesan: 290 calories, 630 mg sodium, 5 g fat, 35 g carbs, 26 g protein, 4 g fiber
- Picante Chicken and Pasta: 260 calories, 480 mg sodium, 4 g fat, 32 g carbs, 23 g protein, 4 g fiber

SOUTH BEACH LIVING

- Kung Pao Chicken: 250 calories, 630 mg sodium, 9 g fat, 14 g carbs, 25 g protein, 4 g fiber
- Chicken Santa Fe Style Rice and Beans: 340 calories, 750 mg sodium, 12 g fat, 35 g carbs, 22 g protein, 4 g fiber

Breads and Cereals

AS I DISCUSSED ON pages 36–37 and pages 56–57, to find whole-grain foods on your supermarket shelves, it's important to read the ingredient listing on the back of the package. If one of the first few ingredients is a whole grain, you are probably holding a whole-grain product in your hands. (Words that indicate whole grains in the ingredients are: 100% whole-wheat flour, brown rice, whole oats or oatmeal, wild rice, whole rye, quinoa, etc.)

Additionally, you can find whole-grain foods by looking for the Whole Grains Council stamp on the package.

Breads

Some grocery stores are beginning to carry high-fiber breads. (By "high-fiber" I mean that they have at least 5 grams of fiber per slice.) You can always find whole-grain, high-fiber bread at a health food store, but here are some of my recommendations for safely navigating the bread aisle at the supermarket:

- Arnold Double Fiber 100% Whole Wheat
- Earth Grains Whole Wheat Bread
- Ezekiel 4:9 bread
- Nature's Own Double Fiber Wheat Bread
- Orowheat Double Fiber Bread
- Sahara Whole Wheat Pita Bread
- Sara Lee Heart Healthy Plus with honey
- Manna Bread

What's in a Name?

Don't assume that different products with the same brand name are all whole grain. You have to read the ingredients list for each different bread variety to be sure. For example: Pepperidge Farm 100% Whole Wheat bread is whole grain, but Pepperidge Farm Light Style 7-Grain bread isn't.

EAT THIS AND LIVE!

Oatmeal

One of the healthiest cereals has been around for years: oatmeal. But again, watch that you don't pick up a man-made "dead" version of this heart-healthy breakfast staple. Steel-cut oatmeal is best, and old-fashioned oatmeal is also fine. However, avoid instant oatmeal and flavored oatmeal because they are processed and have sugars and preservatives added.

Cereals

I describe a product as a "healthy cereal" if it is higher in fiber and lower in sugar content. I recommend that your cereal contain at least 4 grams of fiber and no more than 10 grams of sugar per serving. Here are a few that I feel qualify as healthy:

Pumpernickel

Pumpernickel bread is a great alternative to wheat bread because it usually contains 80 to 90 percent hulled and cracked rye kernels. Rye kernel bread is also an alternative.

- All-Bran, All-Bran Complete Wheat Flakes, and All-Bran Extra Fiber
- Ezekiel 4:9 Whole Grain Flourless Cereal, Original (and all Ezekiel 4:9 cereal varieties)
- Fiber One Caramel Delight
- Kashi Vive, Heart to Heart, and other Kashi cereals
- Nature's Path Organic cereals
- New England Muesli
- Publix Greenwise Flax Flakes
- Quaker Oat Bran
- Steel-cut or old-fashioned oatmeal

Breakfast Cereal or Breakfast Candy?

After analyzing twenty-seven common breakfast cereals, *Consumer Reports* found that eleven of them contain as much sugar as a glazed doughnut. Post Golden Crisp and Kellogg's Honey Smacks ranked worst, containing more than 50 percent sugar. Four cereals were found to have relatively low sugar content and higher levels of dietary fiber: Cheerios, Kix, Life, and Honey Nut Cheerios.[4] Stick with these four cereals or one of the healthier cereals I've recommended on this page.

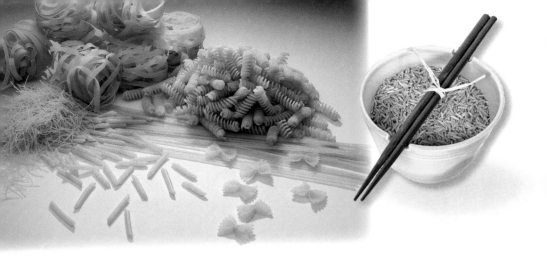

Pastas and Rice

IN ADDITION TO LOOKING for whole-grain products, there are three things to keep in mind when selecting the healthiest pasta possible:

1. MILLING PROCESS: A finely ground grain has a higher glycemic zone value than coarsely ground grain, which has a higher fiber content. Thicker spaghetti has a lower glycemic index than angel hair pasta.
2. COOKING: Most pasta can be either high-glycemic or low-glycemic, depending on how you cook it. If you cook pasta al dente, leaving it firm to the bite, it typically has a low-glycemic value. If the pasta is cooked for a longer period of time and is very soft, it has a high-glycemic value.

Dr. Colbert Approved

Spaghetti Dinner

Cook 4 ounces of whole-wheat spaghetti noodles (not angel hair) according to package directions for al dente (usually five to six minutes). Brown 2–6 ounces of extra-lean organic or free-range beef with chopped onion and a tablespoon of roasted minced garlic. Sprinkle (salt-free and non-irradiated) Italian seasoning and granulated garlic over ground beef while browning. Add salt and pepper to taste. Add Classico Organic Tomato, Herbs & Spices pasta sauce and simmer over low heat until pasta is done cooking. Serve with soup and salad. Makes one serving.

3. PROTEIN CONTENT:
   The higher the protein content of a food, the more it helps prevent a rapid rise in blood sugar and makes the food more likely to be lower glycemic.

I recommend the following brands:

- A company called Eden has a whole line of organic 100 percent whole-grain pastas. Visit their Web site at www.edenfoods.com. You can skip the store and do all of your shopping right from their Web site.

- Westbrae Natural offers organic whole-wheat spaghetti and lasagna noodles.

CAUTION: bottled pasta sauces

Be careful when shopping for pasta sauces. Many of them contain high-fructose corn syrup and other forms of sugar. Choose organic varieties and try to keep the sugar as low as possible. I recommend Classico Organic Tomato, Herbs & Spices.

Other good choices are Muir Glen Organic Portabello Mushroom Sauce and Newman's Own organic sauces, which come in several flavors.

Brown rice and beyond

As I did with breads, I'm challenging you to go beyond whole grains and consider a "sprouted" option. Germinated brown rice is brown rice that is soaked in water, allowing tiny sprouts to grow from the grain. This softens the rice, making it less chewy than regular brown rice and giving it good flavor-absorbing characteristics. At the same time, the germination process enhances the bioavailability of amino acids, vitamins, and minerals. Here are two Web sites where you can find germinated brown rice products: www.SolGrains.com and www.dhccare.com.

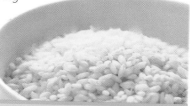

Pasta Portion Distortion

Twenty years ago, a typical restaurant serving of spaghetti and meatballs contained one cup of pasta with sauce and three small meatballs, totaling 500 calories. Today, the same "regular" serving is twice that amount and averages 1,025 calories.[6]

SALAD DRESSINGS, OILS, AND FATS

IT IS BEST TO choose light dressings or one part extra-virgin olive oil with four parts vinegar (balsamic or apple cider vinegar) in a salad spray or spritzer. There are some healthy choices, such as Newman's Own salad dressings. Here are a few more that I can recommend:

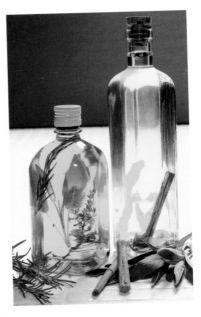

Blue cheese

- Litehouse Lite Blue Cheese Dressing

Caesar

- Cain's Light Caesar Dressing
- Wish-Bone Just 2 Good Light Caesar Dressing

Ranch

- Cain's Light Ranch dressing
- Wish-Bone Just 2 Good Light Ranch Dressing

Thousand Island

- Wish-Bone Just 2 Good Light Thousand Island Dressing

Caesar Savvy

Though a few low-fat choices exist, be extra careful when buying Caesar dressing. The notorious fat-laden dressing is often the worst choice on the condiment aisle. Brands like Ken's Steak House (which contains 9 grams of fat and 80 calories per tablespoon) often tack a "0 g carbs" label on their products. A better choice: Wish-Bone's Caesar Delight Vinaigrette Salad Spritzer, which packs only 2 calories and minimal fat per spray.

Of course, my favorite oil is extra-virgin olive oil. You may also choose other types of oils, but make sure they are cold-expeller pressed vegetable or nut oils. Just remember, even though these are healthy oils, they are still loaded with calories—approximately 120 calories per tablespoon. So go easy on the oil. Here are some tips to help you keep on the light side of oils:

1. Use a healthy oil spray for cooking. Many cooking oils have up to 120 calories per tablespoon, which makes it easy to rack up the calories when using oil to cook or as a salad dressing. I recommend using healthy oils such as extra-virgin olive oil in a spray bottle. You can also stir-fry with a minimum amount of oil.

2. Use a mister with salad dressings to decrease the amount you use. A one-second spray typically contains only about 7 calories. Misters can be found at most cookware stores, and some dressing manufacturers are beginning to sell their products in misters.

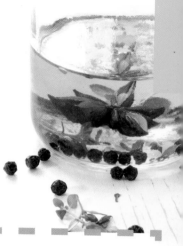

Dr. Colbert Approved

Healthy Fats

Here's what I consider a single serving of healthy fat:

- Almond butter— 2 tablespoons

- Almonds—about 18 almonds

- Avocado, fresh— ½ cup, puréed

- Butter—1 tablespoon

- Cashew butter—2 tablespoons

- Flaxseeds—3 tablespoons

- Smart Balance Light Mayonnaise— 2 tablespoons

- Smart Beat Fat-Free Mayonnaise—up to 5 tablespoons (best to use less)

- Oil (extra-virgin olive oil, extra-virgin coconut oil, or any other healthy oil)—1 tablespoon

- Macadamia nuts—1 ounce

- Pecans—½ ounce

- Pumpkin seeds—¼ cup

- Sunflower seeds—3 tablespoons

- Walnuts—½ ounce

CONDIMENTS

THERE ARE A FEW companies that make condiments with low sugar and healthy ingredients. Visit http://www.westbrae.com/products/condiments.php for some ketchup and mustard products. For a healthier alternative to soy sauce, I recommend Bragg's Liquid Aminos (visit www.bragg.com). Bragg's uses non-GMO soybeans and only has a small amount of naturally occurring sodium. No table salt is added. You can lower your sodium intake even further by diluting Bragg's Liquid Aminos with water before adding it to your recipe or spraying it on your food.

Another option is making your own condiments from scratch to avoid all of the sugars and additives found in store-bought brands. Here are a few recipes I've used in my books over the years.

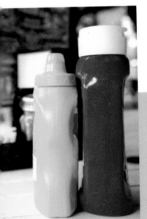

Ketchup[7]

1 cup Westbrae Unsweetened Un-Ketchup

1/16 tsp. pure stevia powder

Mix to combine ingredients. Use as you would regular ketchup. Serves 4.

Mock Sour Cream[8]

1 cup plain low-fat yogurt or Greek-style yogurt

1 tsp. 100 percent pure vegetable glycerine

Mix to combine ingredients. Chill at least 30 minutes before serving. Makes approximately 1 cup.

Nut Butter[9]

½ cup pecans, walnuts, or almonds

1 Tbsp. cold-pressed grapeseed oil

Combine nuts and oil in food processor or blender until creamy. Spread on whole grain bread or use in recipes. Makes ½ cup.

Additive-Free Baking Powder[12]

⅓ cup baking soda

⅔ cup crème of tartar

⅔ cup arrowroot

Mix to combine ingredients. Store and use as you would baking powder. Makes 1⅔ cups.

Cocktail Sauce[10]

1 cup Westbrae Unsweetened Un-Ketchup

¹⁄₁₆ tsp. pure stevia powder

½ tsp. Bragg's Amino Acids

1 Tbsp. organic horseradish (use more or less, according to taste)

Mix to combine ingredients. Garnish with fresh herbs. Serves 6.

Pico de Gallo[13]

2½ cups fresh tomatoes, diced

1 cup onion, diced

½ cup cilantro, chopped

½ cup Serrano peppers, minced

Pinch of sea salt

Squeeze of lemon juice

Mix to combine ingredients. Chill and serve as a condiment. Makes 3½ cups.

Salt-Free Chili Powder[11]

2 Tbsp. paprika

2 tsp. oregano

1¼ tsp. ground cumin

1¼ tsp. garlic powder

¾ tsp. cayenne pepper

¾ tsp. onion powder

Mix to combine ingredients. Store in airtight container. Makes ¼ cup.

Snacks

I ADVISE MY PATIENTS to eat three healthy meals a day, supported by a midafternoon snack. On occasion, you may eat a light evening snack before bed—correctly balanced with proteins, carbohydrates, and fats. A healthy bedtime snack helps to stabilize blood sugar during the night. Here's a list of snack foods I recommend.

Snack bars

- FitSmart Bar (Cranberry Apple, Lemon Poppy, Chocolate Chunk)
- Fiber One (Oats and Chocolate Chewy Bar, Oats and Peanut Butter Chewy Bar)
- Newman's Own food bars

Crackers and cheese
(combine any serving of crackers with any serving of cheese listed here)

- Triscuit Roasted Garlic—1 ounce
- Triscuit Herb Garden—1 ounce
- Triscuit Deli-Style—1 ounce
- Healthy Way Rice Bran—1 ounce
- Kraft Singles Sharp Cheddar, fat-free—two slices, ¾ ounce each
- Kraft Singles American, fat-free—two slices, ¾ ounce each
- Kraft Singles Mozzarella, nonfat—two slices, ¾ ounce each
- Kraft Singles Swiss, nonfat—two slices, ¾ ounce each
- Breakstone Cottage Cheese, nonfat—½ cup

Kefir and fruit smoothie
Blend 6 to 8 ounces of Lifeway organic, low-fat, plain kefir and one medium apple. You may add 1 or 2 tablespoons of ground flaxseeds.

Cheese, fruit, and nuts

- Two slices of organic fat-free cheese, one medium organic apple, and five to ten pecans, walnuts, or almonds

Protein powder shake
Blend one scoop of powdered whey or rice protein with 8 ounces of organic skim milk or rice milk and 1 to 2 tablespoons of ground flaxseeds. You may also add ¼ cup of berries or half of a banana.

Bedtime Snacks

For a quick fix that won't keep you up all night, try these:

- A piece of fruit, like a small apple, grapefruit, 4 ounces of berries or kiwi, with a small handful of nuts (walnuts, almonds, or pecans)

- One serving of low-fat, whole-grain crackers or one piece of whole-grain bread with about a teaspoon of organic almond butter or two ounces of turkey

- One-half cup organic skim milk or low-fat cottage cheese or low-fat, no-sugar kefir or yogurt (if not sensitive to dairy) with fruit added

- A small bowl of whole-grain cereal (about ¼ to ½ cup) with organic skim milk

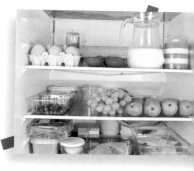

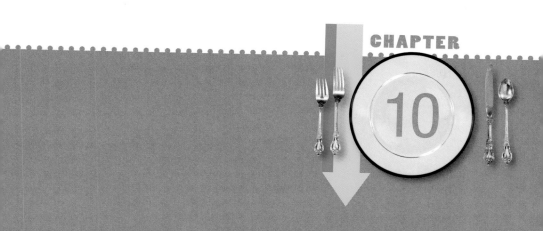

DINNER'S READY!— HOW TO STORE, PREPARE, AND SERVE FOOD

DON'T IGNORE IT, STORE IT!

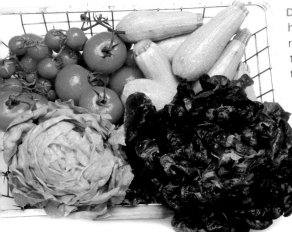

DINNER SHOULD BE THE most pleasant hour of your day, a time to slow down, relax, and gather with family and friends to enjoy food and fellowship. Here are tips for keeping food healthy all the way to the dinner table. I admit that extra effort is required on your part for healthy storage of food. But I assure you that it is well worth it once you realize both the immediate and long-term benefits for not only you but also your family.

Food Storage Tips

Here are some quick tips for storing foods as safely as possible and avoiding nutrient loss:

- Start purchasing foods that are the highest quality and the most recently harvested. (Organic, locally grown foods are best.)

- If you can, buy your food the day you intend to eat it, or a day or two before. This means buying in smaller quantities so you consume everything quickly.

- If you overestimate and buy more than you can use, freezing produce before it sits around for days is an option, but fresh is still best.

- Refrigerate your produce below 40 degrees to avoid vitamin loss.

- Keep frozen foods below 0 degrees to retain maximum vitamin content.

- Separate fruits that ripen (plums, peppers, etc.) from root crops and leafy greens in your refrigerator. Root crops do best when they are stored somewhere cool and moist; leafy greens (spinach, broccoli, salad greens, etc.) keep their nutrients best when stored in high humidity; fresh veggies and fruits retain the most nutrients when stored at the coldest possible temperature without freezing.

- Don't chop your food ahead of time, as damaging the tissues of the produce speeds up nutrient loss.

- Be aware of which nutrients are most sensitive, such as vitamin C, which is sensitive to air, light, and heat during storage. (See sidebar on the facing page for more information.)

How Long Do Fresh Foods Retain Their Nutrients?

Some people buy fresh fruits and vegetables and store them for days and weeks before using them. They assume that as long as the produce looks or tastes good, it is safe to keep it around. However, the longer the food is stored, the more vitamin and phytonutrient content is lost. (There is one ray of sunshine: Kathleen Brown, professor of postharvest physiology, says that while vitamins and phytonutrients decline, mineral nutrients will not change at all.[1])

Grapes can lose a third of their B vitamins, and tangerines can lose up to half of their vitamin C if left on the counter for a long time. Asparagus stored for one week can lose 90 percent of its vitamin C.

Temperature seems to have the greatest impact on *senescence*, the process in which enzymes break down the food on a cellular level. Luke LaBorde, associate professor of food science at Penn State University, found that spinach stored at 39 degrees Fahrenheit loses its folate and carotenoid content at a slower rate than spinach stored at 50 and 68 degrees.

Although keeping fresh foods cool is a start, the clock is still ticking. Even at 39 degrees, LaBorde's spinach retained only 53 percent of its folate after eight days.[2]

Stability of Various Nutrients in Storage[3]

Nutrient	Stability
Vitamin A	Sensitive to air, light, and heat
Vitamin C*	Sensitive to air, light, and heat
Vitamin D	Somewhat sensitive to air, light, and heat
Thiamin*	Sensitive to air and heat
Folic acid*	Sensitive to air, light, and heat
Vitamin K	Somewhat sensitive to air and light
Vitamin B_6	Sensitive to light and heat
Riboflavin	Sensitive to light and heat
Biotin, Niacin	Relatively stable
Carotenes	Sensitive to air, light, and heat
*These nutrients are most unstable	

Nutrients Lost in Frozen Foods

Freezing meat can destroy up to 50 percent of thiamin and riboflavin and 70 percent of pantothenic acids, so fresh is always best.

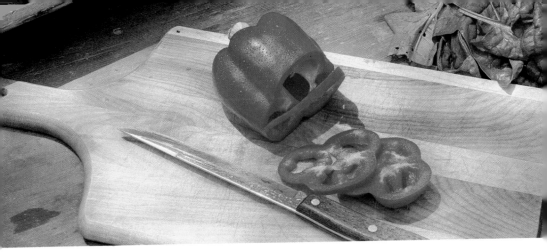

PREPARATION

RECENT OUTBREAKS OF FOOD-BORNE illness associated with produce such as spinach and tomatoes have received widespread media and public attention. As a result, consumers have a heightened concern for the safety of these fresh foods. While there's nothing you can do to avoid recalls of foods that are contaminated during commercial growing, harvesting, or processing, there are ways to make sure you don't add to the risk of food contamination by following proper food preparation safety tips at home.

The FDA and other government organizations offer tons of food safety tips at www.foodsafety.gov. On the facing page, I've listed a few tips I consider essential when handling and preparing fresh foods.

Antibacterial Solutions

Dr. Colbert Approved

For the best bacteria protection, I recommend a diluted bleach mixture (1 Tbsp. Clorox bleach to 1 gal. water). For surfaces that come in contact with food, you must use Clorox regular bleach and not a generic brand that may contain additional chemicals. Store this diluted Clorox in a spray bottle under the sink for easy access. Clorox disinfecting wipes are an even more convenient solution, and I recommend them as well.

If you prefer natural options for sanitizing your kitchen, some very effective natural antibacterial agents are white vinegar, grapefruit seed extract, orange peel extract, or tea tree oil.

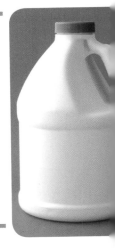

- Always wash your hands before handling fresh foods, and wash them often during preparation.

- Wash produce in cool water to remove dirt and pesticide residues.

- Be sure the surface of your prep station and cutting boards have been washed with hot water and soap or antibacterial cleansers. (See the sidebar on the previous page for my recommended antibacterial solutions.)

- Keep your foods separated at the grocery store. (Place raw meats in plastic bags to keep leaking juices from contaminating other foods in your grocery cart.) Continue to separate foods during home storage and meal preparation to avoid cross-contamination. One way to do this is to use different cutting boards and utensils for fresh produce and raw meat. Wash your hands after handling raw meat, and place the cutting board and any dishes and utensils that touched the raw meat into the sink to be washed with hot, soapy water.

- Use separate utensils for handling raw and cooked foods. Don't use the same spoon, spatula, or set of tongs to transfer raw food to the stove or oven that you use to transfer cooked food from the stove or oven to the table.

- Never place cooked food back on the same plate that it sat on when it was raw.

- Marinate foods in the refrigerator, not on the counter.

- Defrost frozen foods in the refrigerator, not on the counter. Never refreeze defrosted foods.

- Never leave refrigerated foods at room temperature for more than two hours. (Limit this to one hour if it's a hot day.)

Sometimes It's Better to Procrastinate!

I always advise people to wash, cut, and prepare fruits or vegetables just before you are ready to eat them. It's tempting to slice them up early for the sake of convenience, but once exposed to air, they begin to lose nutrients like vitamin C, folic acid, vitamin B_{12}, biotin, and vitamins D, E, K, and A. If you must chop or cut up your vegetables, do so just before eating them when the nutritional value will still be high.

The same goes for cooking food. Though busy homemakers like to prepare meals in advance, keep in mind that reheating food and leftovers depletes them of vitamins, minerals, and nutrients. A fresh-made dish is more nutritious than one you cook and refrigerate.

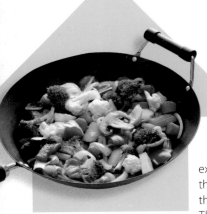

HEALTHY COOKING

I RECOMMEND SEVERAL DIFFERENT cooking methods on these pages, as well as warning you about unhealthy cooking methods to avoid. Most importantly, whatever cooking method you use, remember not to kill living foods by over-cooking them. Researcher Edward Howell devoted nearly his entire life to researching enzymes. He found that when food is cooked at temperatures exceeding 118 degrees for thirty minutes, almost all the enzymes are destroyed. These enzymes are the living part of the food.[4]

When you boil vegetables, the nutrients leach into the water. By the time the vegetables are tender enough to eat, the mineral and vitamin content of the water is greater than that of the vegetables! You have created a dead food from a living food.

If you must boil vegetables, bring the water to a boil first, and then add your vegetables for a brief time. Do not allow them to soak in the water. Drain them immediately and serve them. If possible, just quit boiling vegetables altogether.

Never deep-fry foods. The oils used in deep-frying are usually toxic and the meat soaks up these harmful oils like a sponge. However, light stir-frying in healthy oils is acceptable.

The Best—and Worst—Oils for Cooking

Here's a list of the best—and worst—cooking oils, from high to low smoke point.[5] (As I mentioned on page 63, the lower the smoke point, the quicker the oil breaks down to create free radicals.)

Best	Smoke Point (Fahrenheit)	Worst	Smoke Point (Fahrenheit)
Rice bran oil	495 degrees	Lard	370 degrees
Grapeseed oil	420 degrees	Corn oil, unrefined	320 degrees
Macadamia nut oil	390 degrees	Soy oil, unrefined	320 degrees
Butter	350 degrees	Safflower oil, unrefined	225 degrees
Coconut oil	350 degrees	Canola, unrefined	225 degrees
Extra-virgin olive oil	320 degrees		

Wave Good-bye to the Microwave

One study found that just six minutes of microwave cooking destroyed half the vitamin B_{12} in dairy foods and meat, a much higher rate of destruction than other cooking methods.[6] In another test, microwaved broccoli lost between 87 and 97 percent of several major cancer-protecting antioxidants.[7] I recommend using a convection oven or a toaster oven to heat up just about anything that you would heat in a microwave oven.

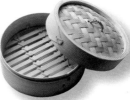

Dr. Colbert Approved

Cooking Methods

➤ STIR-FRY. Use a little bit of organic coconut oil, organic butter, ghee (clarified butter), or macadamia nut oil. Extra-virgin olive oil has a lower smoke point than these oils and will begin to break down when heated over 320 degrees Fahrenheit.

➤ STEAMING. This is a wonderful way to cook vegetables. *Lightly* steaming your vegetables causes very little loss of nutrients.

➤ GRILLING. Use a propane gas grill in place of charcoal or mesquite, which contain dangerous chemicals. Place the meat rack as high as possible, away from the flame. When meat cooks over a flame, fat drips into the fire and turns into steam. The pesticides in the fat char into the meat. Charred meat contains a chemical called benzopyrene, which is a highly carcinogenic substance. Scrape off char. Don't even give it to the dog.

➤ BAKING OR ROASTING. Drizzle or spritz meats and vegetables with olive oil, sea salt, and fresh-ground black pepper. Then roast them in the oven for half an hour, and you have a tasty, healthy alternative to fried foods. Sweet potatoes, tomatoes, and asparagus are especially tasty when roasted this way.

Cookware

I explain in detail the harmfulness of certain types of cookware in my book *The Seven Pillars of Health*. Here's a list of cookware I recommend as healthy:

- Glass bakeware and cookware (Pyrex is excellent)

- Ceramic cookware (CorningWare is a brand I recommend), but throw away if the enamel becomes chipped

- Stainless steel cookware

- Anodized aluminum cookware uses an electro-chemical anodizing process that seals the aluminum, preventing leaching into the food. This is the *only* acceptable option for aluminum cookware.

SETTING THE STAGE FOR DINNER

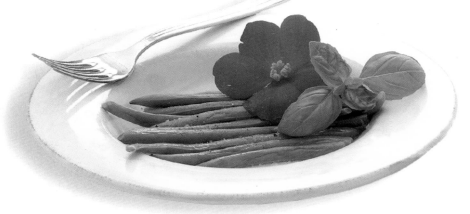

THE ATMOSPHERE AT DINNERTIME should be completely joyful. Turn off the TV. Don't watch sporting events, the news, or suspenseful movies at dinner. Start your meal with a heartfelt blessing. Pause and consider how thankful you are. Then keep the conversation pleasant. Don't use the dinner table as a time to hold court on your children or to bring up troubling topics. Never make dinner a time to reprimand one another or argue. In Leonardo da Vinci's *The Last Supper*, you see the disciples laughing, talking, and leaning against Jesus in complete fellowship. That's a good model.

I sometimes hear people yelling and arguing in restaurants. That is the worst way to eat! When you are stressed, you can't digest well. Blood flows away from the digestive tract to the muscles for a fight-or-flight response. This shuts down the digestive juices. Food stays in the stomach longer, causing heartburn and indigestion. Also, the food is not digested properly, leading to bloating, gas, constipation, and even diarrhea.

If you are upset, angry, or in an irritated mood, wait to eat.

Getting back to eating meals together as a family—even if just one or two days a week—is important, especially for children. Sitting down to a meal together, especially dinner, gives parents a chance to reconnect with their children. Even if they're teenagers, you can attempt to spend time with them. The benefits will extend far beyond nutrition. Studies have found that teens who have five or more family dinners per week are three times less likely to try marijuana, two and a half times less likely to smoke cigarettes, and one and a half times less likely to drink alcohol than those who eat less often with their families. Studies also show that teens who eat with their parents are more likely to get better grades and to know that their parents are proud of them.[8]

Healthy Eating Tips

- Chew each bite at least twenty to thirty times, and put your fork down between bites. Your saliva contains special enzymes called *ptyalin* and *amylase*, which digest carbohydrates. Let these enzymes do their work.

- Use your molars to chew. Don't use your canines to eat, as lions and tigers do. They have short digestive tracts and tremendous levels of hydrochloric acid to break down the meat. By contrast, you and I don't produce enough hydrochloric acid to digest half-chewed meat, so it putrefies in the intestines.

- Slow down and enjoy what you are eating. Rushing through a meal causes hydrochloric acid to be suppressed, making digestion difficult. It also encourages you to eat more than you should. It takes about twenty minutes for your hypothalamus, located in your brain, to tell you that you are full. Many people can shovel in thousands of calories before the hypothalamus finally registers "enough."

- Don't drink cold drinks with food. It dampens and dilutes hydrochloric acid, digestive juices, and enzymes. It's similar to starting a campfire and then pouring water on it. However, a cup of hot organic tea may benefit digestion.

- Eat the protein portion of your meal first since this stimulates glucagon, which will depress insulin secretion and cause the release of carbohydrates that have been stored in the liver and muscles, which will help prevent low blood sugar.

- Limit your starches to only one serving per meal. Never eat bread, pasta, potatoes, corn, and different starches together at one meal. This elevates insulin levels. If you feel like having seconds, choose fruits, vegetables, and salads, not more starches.

- And remember to exercise temperance. Dinner should not be the blowout meal of the day. I tell my patients to eat breakfast like a king, lunch like a prince, and dinner like a pauper. Eat moderate portions and feast instead on conversation and laughter.

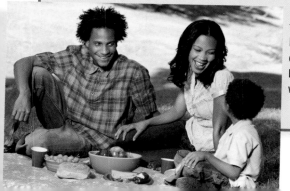

Generally your first deep breath toward the end of a meal is a sign that your body is satisfied and that you should stop eating. Continuing to eat after this deep breath regularly will eventually result in weight gain.

ON THE GO?—
SMART CHOICES
FOR DINING OUT

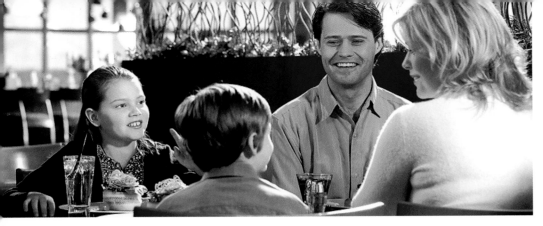

EATING OUT

WE ALL HAVE OUR favorite restaurants, but did you know that some Americans eat almost six meals outside of the home each week? This amounts to more than three hundred meals a year. It's impossible to dine out this often without gaining weight and creating a host of other health problems—unless you commit to sticking with the basic rules of healthy eating.

I've had many patients ask me for advice on ordering healthy food when eating out. When I ask them what they usually eat at restaurants, I discover most of them make wise choices with the dishes they've chosen; however, they either forget about eating smaller portion sizes or neglect to apply the rules to all the extra things that are usually consumed when dining out. You'll rarely be able to order a perfect meal when dining out, but these are the tips I've learned over the years for choosing the healthiest options possible.

- You can order the right meal and still blow it on the beverage. Save hundreds of unneeded calories by passing on the soda when eating out. And don't think the diet soda is any better. It's not—it's worse! Choose fresh-brewed, unsweetened iced tea, hot tea, water, or sparkling water instead.

- Skip the bread.

- Order soup. This will help fill you up and make it easier to avoid the unhealthy temptations that accompany your main course and dessert. Make sure to stick to broth-based soups such as chicken and wild rice, vegetable, or bean soup, rather than cream-based soups like broccoli and cheddar.

- Request romaine lettuce instead of iceberg lettuce when you order salad. And ask for olive oil and vinegar as a dressing (in a mister, if available) rather than high-fat, high-sugar prepared salad dressings. Remember to order a salad with a variety of fruits, vegetables, seeds, and nuts that give you the full rainbow of colorful phytonutrient power.

- Order whole-wheat buns or pasta whenever possible. More and more restaurants are making these healthy substitutions available. Some Asian restaurants are beginning to offer brown rice as an alternative to white rice or fried rice. No more than a tennis-ball sized portion of any pasta or rice should be consumed.

- When your entrée arrives, don't fall into the trap of feeling like you have to eat everything on your plate. Most restaurant portions are much too large. A healthy portion size for most men is about 4 oz. of lean protein like steak, chicken, or turkey, and for most women a healthy portion is about 3 oz.

- Choose a main entrée that you and your spouse or companion would both like to eat, and split it.

- Try to make at least half of your total meal consist of fresh fruits and vegetables. If you are at a buffet and want to go back for seconds,

visit the salad bar for more fruits and veggies instead of doubling up on protein and carbs.

- If you crave dessert, try skipping the bread and the carbs in your main entrée (potatoes, rice, pasta, corn, etc.). Or try opting for fruit as a dessert or splitting a dessert order with a few friends.

- Plan what and where you'll eat before heading out, and if possible, eat an early dinner so you can finish your meal early enough to burn off many of the calories before you go to bed.

- Independently owned restaurants are often more flexible with menu substitutions since they are preparing and cooking your food on site and do not have to use prepackaged food items like chain restaurants often do. Keep this in mind as you are choosing where you want to eat.

- Learn healthy food selections from the most common types of restaurants, especially if you know you'll be dining at them

every now and then. Most national chains provide all of their nutritional content on a Web site or as a brochure in the restaurant. Web sites such as www.health ydiningfinder.com are an excellent resource for learning about healthy restaurant choices.

- If you are going to be traveling by car, figure out where you'll be along your route when meal times occur. Then, since fast food tends to be less healthy than other restaurant fare, find out where the nearest sit-down restaurants are in that area. Pack a few healthy snacks like fruits, vegetables, and nuts to hold kids over until you reach your preplanned restaurant, rather than giving in to the temptation to find the nearest drive-through when hunger strikes.

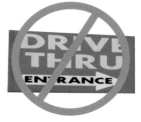

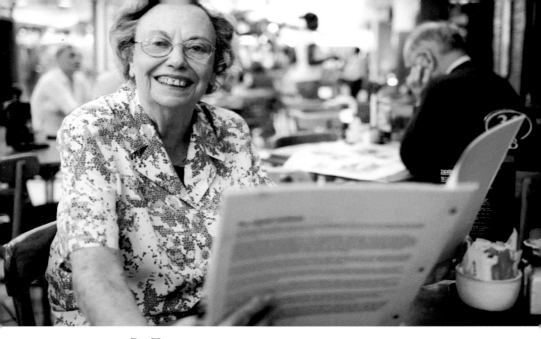

NAVIGATING THE
MENU MAZE

PEOPLE WHO CREATE RESTAURANT menus realize that words like "deep-fried" might turn you off, so they opt for words like "extra crispy" in the moniker instead. Just because sugar, calories, and fat don't show up on the menu, that doesn't mean they don't show up in the food. Knowing which words to watch for can help you avoid unhealthy choices. Here's a rundown of some of the more common terms on restaurant menus. These are just general guidelines. Ask your server questions, and use your best judgment when dining out.

Probably Healthy	Probably Unhealthy
Braised	Au gratin
Broiled	Basted
Dry-aged	Battered
Fresh	Bottomless
Grilled	Breaded
Marinated	Blackened
Reduced	Cheesy
Roasted	Creamy
Sautéed	Crispy
Seared	Crunchy
Seasoned	Deep-fried
Smoked	Endless
Steamed	Glazed
Stir-fried	Loaded
Vegetarian	Smothered
Wilted	Stuffed

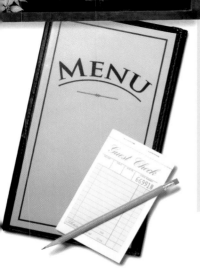

FDA Menu Regulations

You probably knew that the FDA regulates the use of words that describe nutrients in food on labels in the grocery store, but did you know they also regulate the use of these words on restaurant menus? Here are the standard FDA definitions for some common menu lingo:[1]

- **Cholesterol-free:** Food containing less than 2 mg of cholesterol and 2 g or less of saturated fat per serving
- **Fat-free:** Food containing less than 0.5 g of fat per serving
- **Lean:** A serving of meat, poultry, or seafood that contains less than 10 g of fat, 4 g of saturated fat, and 95 mg of cholesterol
- **Light, lite:** Food that has 33 percent less calories, 50 percent less fat, or 50 percent less sodium than what is customarily consumed
- **Low-calorie:** Main dishes containing 100 calories or less per serving
- **Low-fat:** Food containing 3 g of fat or less per serving
- **Low-sodium:** Food containing 140 mg of sodium or less per serving
- **Reduced cholesterol:** Food containing a minimum of 25 percent less cholesterol and 2 g or less of saturated fat per serving than what is customarily consumed
- **Reduced calories:** Food containing a minimum of 25 percent fewer calories per serving than what is customarily consumed
- **Reduced fat:** Food containing a minimum of 25 percent less fat per serving than what is customarily consumed
- **Reduced sodium:** Food containing a minimum of 25 percent less sodium per serving than what is customarily consumed
- **Reduced sugar:** Food containing a minimum of 25 percent less sugar per serving than what is customarily consumed
- **Sugar-free:** Food containing less than 0.5 grams of sugar per serving

Fast-Food Restaurants

FAST-FOOD RESTAURANTS ARE NOT an ideal option for a healthy eating lifestyle. But in the event that this cannot be avoided, try the following at a typical hamburger-oriented fast-food chain:

- Instead of ordering a double cheeseburger (around 700 calories), large french fries (approximately 500 calories), and a large coke (about 300 calories), a healthier choice would be to order a grilled chicken sandwich or a small hamburger.

- Order a whole-grain bun if available.

- If white buns are the only option, throw away the top bun and keep the bottom one. Another option is to cut the sandwich in half and stack both halves of meat between one half of the top and bottom bun.

- Order your burger in a separate container and squeeze it between two napkins to remove excess grease.

- Use mustard, lettuce, tomato, onions, and pickle instead of mayonnaise and ketchup.

- Order a small salad with dressing on the side and a cup of unsweetened iced tea or a bottle of water with lemon.

- Instead of french fries, try a baked potato, if available, using only one pat of butter or two teaspoons of sour cream.

- Remember to never supersize.

Pizza can be one of the worst weight-loss saboteurs of all. Before diving in, eat a large salad with dressing on the side. Choose a thin crust with veggies as toppings. Also, request your pizza with half the cheese and part skim mozzarella. Practice moderation when it comes to any pizza. Never have more than two slices.

Dr. Colbert Approved

Boston Market Menu Items

Quick Tips: No skin, no gravy, and use light salad dressing in place of regular salad dressing. Choose Garlic Dill New Potatoes instead of mashed potatoes, and save 70 calories and 6 g fat.

- 3-piece Dark Rotisserie Chicken, no skin (240 calories, 8 g fat)
- ¼ White Rotisserie Chicken, no skin (210 calories, 2 g fat)
- Roasted Turkey Breast, 5 oz. (180 calories, 3 g fat)

- Market Chopped Salad with Light Ranch Dressing (280 calories, 13 g fat)
- Fresh Steamed Vegetables (60 calories, 2 g fat)
- Green Beans (60 calories, 4 g fat)
- Seasonal Fresh Fruit (60 calories, 0 g fat)

EAT THIS and LIVE!

Chick-fil-A Menu Items

I encourage you to eat at Chick-fil-A because they are one of the healthiest fast-food restaurant chains around (all of their sandwiches are less than 500 calories), and also because Chick-fil-A's founder is a Christian.

- Chargrilled Chicken Cool Wrap (410 calories, 12 g fat)
- Spicy Chicken Cool Wrap (400 calories, 12 g fat)
- Chargrilled Chicken Sandwich (270 calories, 3 g fat)
- Chargrilled Chicken Club Sandwich (380 calories, 11 g fat)

Subway Sandwiches

Make sure you order a 6-inch on wheat bread or pita bread. Hold the mayo and ask for mustard or vinegar and light oil. Values below include wheat bread, lettuce, tomatoes, onion, green peppers, pickles, and olives.

- Ham (290 calories, 5 g fat)
- Oven Roasted Chicken Breast (310 calories, 5 g fat)
- Roast Beef (290 calories, 5 g fat)
- Turkey Breast (280 calories, 4.5 g fat)
- Subway Club (320 calories, 6 g fat)

Quiznos Menu Items

Make sure all sandwiches are small or medium and on wheat bread. Values below reflect small sandwiches on wheat bread with lettuce, tomato, and red onion. Cheese, additional vegetables, and condiments are listed where applicable. Hold the cheese on any item below, and you'll drop about 40–50 calories and 3–4 grams of fat.

- Honey Bourbon Chicken Sub with Honey Bourbon Mustard and Zesty Grille Sauce (320 calories, 4.5 g fat)
- Traditional Sub with Reduced-Fat Buttermilk Ranch Dressing* and cheddar cheese (360 calories, 13 fat)
- Turkey Ranch and Swiss Sub with Reduced-Fat Buttermilk Ranch Dressing* (340 calories, 10 g fat)

  * This dressing requires a special request.

BUFFET-STYLE RESTAURANTS, SALAD BARS, STEAK HOUSES, AND SEAFOOD

Buffets and salad bars

Like fast-food restaurants, buffet-style restaurants should be avoided. Most buffets are loaded with fried foods, unhealthy starches, and a wide assortment of fattening desserts. These restaurants offer too much food and too few wise choices, with the exception of some salads and vegetables.

There are, of course, a few alternatives for the all-you-can-eat variety. Healthier buffets such as the local country club Sunday buffet can actually be a good choice. These buffets often offer beautiful salads, fruits, vegetables, smoked salmon, lean meats, fish, and grilled or baked chicken.

If you find yourself at a buffet-style restaurant, the best way to stay healthy is to simply start with a large salad and fruit, followed by an entrée with plenty of vegetables. Usually by eating plenty of these healthy foods you may not desire a dessert or will only want a bite or two.

Dr. Colbert Approved

Sweet Tomatoes

Sweet Tomatoes is a buffet-style restaurant that provides fresh, whole foods. Their 55-foot salad bar is full of garden-fresh salads, fruits, and vegetables. Right now, you can find Sweet Tomatoes in about fifteen states, and hopefully this healthy buffet option will make its way to more states soon. As with all buffets, the temptation is to overeat. Keep in mind that the values shown are based on a serving size of 1 cup.

The following fresh-tossed salads all have between 120–150 calories and 6–9 grams of fat:

- Classic Greek
- Ensalada Azteca With Turkey
- Honey Minted Fruit Toss
- Roma Tomato
- Mozzarella and Basil
- Strawberry Fields With Carmelized Walnuts

The following prepared salads all have between 140–260 calories and 0–6 grams of fat:

- Aunt Doris' Red Pepper Slaw
- Marinated Summer Vegetables
- Carrot Raisin
- Mandarin Noodles With Broccoli and Sesame Seeds
- Oriental Ginger Slaw With Krab
- Penne Pasta With Chicken in a Citrus Vinaigrette
- Southern Dill Potato
- Southwestern Rice and Beans
- Spicy Southwestern Pasta
- Summer Barley With Black Beans
- Confetti Avocado Slaw

Steak and seafood

These restaurants are common choices to celebrate special occasions. Here are a few general guidelines to keep you on the straight and narrow while dining at these restaurants.

➤ Portion sizes are always large and should be split between two people. This includes the baked potato, of which you should only eat half with one pat of butter or 1 to 2 teaspoons of sour cream and chives.

➤ Ask your server to either hold the bread until the main entrée or skip it altogether.

➤ Choose a lean, petite fillet. You can also order grilled or baked chicken or grilled fish.

➤ Choose steamed vegetables and a large salad, and ask for low-fat or light salad dressing on the side so you can control how much you consume. (Request a salad mister, if available.)

➤ Beware of béarnaise sauce, hollandaise sauce, gravies, creamed vegetables, cheese sauce, and au gratin dishes since they are loaded with fat.

Dr. Colbert Approved

EAT THIS AND LIVE!

Outback Steakhouse

Your healthiest options at any steak house are going to be the seafood menu items and salads. However, if you're really in the mood for a steak, I recommend a meal consisting of the following items from the Outback menu. Remember two things: (1) This portion of meat is enough to split in half, and (2) never order items like the Cheesy Fries (2,900 calories) or the Bloomin' Onion (2,310 calories)!

• Herb Rubbed Slow-Roasted Sirloin, 9 oz. (394 calories, 26 g fat)
• Green Beans (40 calories, 0.1 g fat)
• Whole Grain Wild Rice or Sweet Potato (225 calories, 9.7 g fat)

Red Lobster

When prepared healthily, seafood can be one of the best choices for eating right. If you live near the ocean, as I do in Florida, seafood restaurants with freshly caught menu options abound. However, to give you some healthy options from a national restaurant chain, I recommend the following from Red Lobster. Choose broccoli and whole-grain rice as your sides (no cheddar biscuits!) with any of these menu options:

• Grilled or broiled fresh tilapia* (346 calories, 10 g fat)
• Broiled Flounder (240 calories, 5 g fat)
• Grilled Chicken Breast (314 calories, 8 g fat)

 * Availability based on location

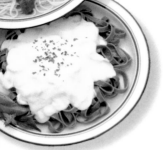

ITALIAN AND MEXICAN RESTAURANTS

Italian restaurants

Italian restaurants are my favorites, but like you, I have to guard against unhealthy options. Here are my guidelines:

➤ Start with a non-cream based soup, such as minestrone or pasta fagioli.

➤ Have a large salad with low-fat or light salad dressing on the side or use a salad mister, if available.

➤ Be especially careful with the bread—even if it's served with olive oil for dipping. People think olive oil is healthy, and it is. But remember, olive oil has 120 calories per tablespoon, and those calories can add up quickly if you are mindlessly eating a whole loaf of bread while waiting for your entrée to arrive.

➤ Grilled chicken, fish, shellfish, veal, or steak is usually a good option.

➤ Avoid fried dishes or Parmesan dishes.

➤ Have your vegetables steamed, and ask that they be prepared without butter.

➤ Ask for whole-grain pasta when available, and ask that it be cooked al dente. (Remember, the thicker the pasta is, the lower it ranks on the glycemic index scale.) Don't overdo it; you should only consume the size of a tennis ball. Take the rest home for another meal.

➤ Avoid creamy sauces, cheese, and pesto sauce since they are loaded with fat.

Dr. Colbert Approved

Olive Garden
- Apricot Chicken (328 calories, 7 g fat)
- Venetian Apricot Chicken (448 calories, 11 g fat)

Romano's Macaroni Grill
- Pollo Magro "Skinny Chicken" (410 calories, 6 g fat)

Mexican and Tex-Mex restaurants

I have found ways to enjoy eating at Mexican restaurants by choosing fajitas with chicken. I find that fajitas are a healthier option because the meat is usually stir-fried or grilled. You can also add fresh ingredients like salsa, tomatoes, onions, lettuce, black beans, pinto beans (not refried), and guacamole. Here are few more general guidelines:

➤ Avoid or limit considerably the chips unless they are baked; still, I caution you not to overeat. A serving is 17–19 chips.

➤ Tortilla soup (without the tortilla chips) and black bean soup are good appetizer selections.

➤ If salad is available, enjoy a large one with low-fat dressing in a salad mister, if available, before your meal.

➤ Opt for fresh salsa, pico de gallo, or low-fat dressing on your salad.

➤ Avoid anything that is topped with melted cheese.

➤ Beware of sour cream—avoid it altogether unless your restaurant serves a low-fat variety.

➤ Go easy on the rice or avoid it altogether since it is usually not whole grain. Like pasta, you should not consume more than a tennis-ball-sized portion.

➤ Some restaurants now offer whole-wheat tortillas; choose only one or two of these if available, or even better, wrap your fajita in a large piece of lettuce instead. Remember to choose only one starch (either rice or tortillas) even when it is whole grain.

Dr. Colbert Approved

Chipotle Mexican Grill

Chipotle Mexican Grill uses naturally raised meats that are free of antibiotics and growth hormones. To save calories and carbs, opt for your burrito or fajita in a bowl instead of wrapped in a flour tortilla. Or ask for a salad and get leafy romaine lettuce instead of rice. You can order many different ways and still have a healthy meal, but only add a little cheese or low-fat sour cream to your order. Here are two healthy options:

- Sample Fajita Bowl: Chicken, rice, lettuce, and salsa (385 calories, 15 g fat)
- Sample Burrito Bowl: Chicken, rice, black beans, corn, and salsa (489 calories, 18 g fat)

ASIAN RESTAURANTS

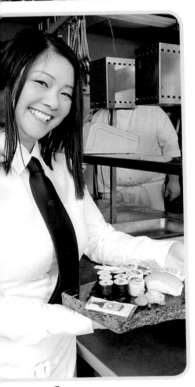

Chinese, Thai, or Vietnamese restaurants

These are usually good choices, provided your meat or seafood is baked, steamed, poached, or stir-fried. Steaming is usually the healthiest method of cooking in Chinese restaurants. Be aware that some Chinese restaurants stir-fry their meat in excessive oil and may use as much as a half a cup of oil to cook your food. Ask them to use minimal oil when stir-frying your meal. Remember that eating white rice is like eating sugar. Here are a few general guidelines for healthier options:

- Instead of fried rice or fried noodles, choose brown rice if available.

- Substitute your serving of rice with vegetables.

- If brown rice or vegetable substitutions are not available, eat no more than the size of a tennis ball of rice.

- Sweet and sour, batter-fried, or twice-cooked food should be avoided since they are generally high in fat and calories.

- Avoid oily sauces such as duck sauce.

- For an appetizer, you can choose wonton or egg drop soup.

- Avoid egg rolls since they are deep-fried and extremely high in fat.

⚠ A Word of Caution About Soy Sauce

A single tablespoon of soy sauce contains more than four times the RDA of sodium. Make sure to use the low-sodium variety, and even then, use it sparingly.

Japanese restaurants

Japanese food is usually low in fat and provides many vegetables. Unfortunately, it is also high in sodium, mainly because of the abundant use of soy sauce. An easy solution to this is to add only a small amount of additional soy sauce (if any) to your food. Here are a few more general guidelines:

- Sushi is fine, and some restaurants even prepare it with brown rice.

- Steamed vegetables, vegetable soups, and salads with dressing on the side are also good choices.

- Seafood, chicken, and beef can be cooked teriyaki style.

- Fish can be steamed or poached.

- Be cautious with eating too much rice, and avoid fried foods.

MSG Warning

The downside of many Chinese restaurants is that they use monosodium glutamate (MSG) to enhance the flavors of most of their main dishes. I strongly recommend that you find a restaurant that doesn't use MSG or at least is willing to not use it on your dishes. MSG has numerous potential reactions. (See pages 30–31 for more information on MSG.)

PF Chang's

- Buddha's Feast Steamed (230 calories, 2 g fat) TIP: If served with tofu, I recommend that you ask them to leave this out.
- Oriental Chicken Salad, dressing not included (450 calories, 10 g fat)
- Oolong Marinated Sea Bass (520 calories, 12 g fat)

Dr. Colbert Approved

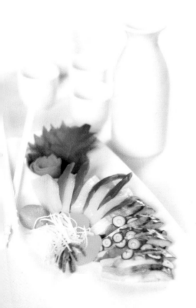

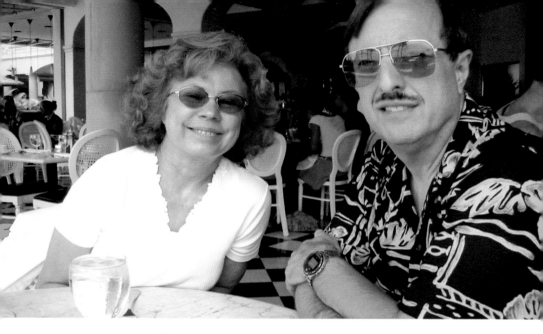

Casual Dining

THESE RESTAURANTS ARE TYPICALLY high in fats, and the main courses are usually fried. The vegetables are usually loaded with gravy, butter, or oil. Good choices include baked or grilled chicken, turkey, or beef with steamed vegetables. Vegetable soup and a salad (with salad dressing on the side) are also good choices. Avoid the large dinner rolls with butter, as well as any fried side dishes. Choose any beans, including lima beans, pinto beans, or string beans. If you must have gravy, have it served on the side and eat sparingly. Although I was raised on Southern cooking, I have learned to still enjoy the foods without all the gravies and fried coatings.

If you enjoy a good barbecue restaurant, keep these general guidelines in mind:

- No skin on your chicken
- Use barbecue sauce sparingly
- Choose corn as a side dish or a tennis-ball-sized serving of baked beans
- Skip the bread
- Order a salad with low-fat or light dressing on the side

On the next three pages, you'll see a number of restaurants I consider family-style, casual dining, and my picks for the healthiest fare.

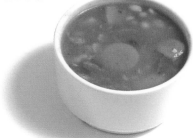

Applebee's

- Grilled Chili-Lime Chicken Salad (250 calories, 6 g fat)
- Cajun Lime Tilapia (310 calories, 6 g fat)
- Steak & Portobellos (330 calories, 10 g fat)
- Italian Chicken & Portobello Sandwich (360 calories, 6 g fat)
- Garlic Herb Chicken (370 calories, 6 g fat)
- Tortilla Chicken Melt (480 calories, 13 g fat)

Chili's

- Grilled Caribbean Salad (440 calories, 10 g fat)
- Chicken Fajita Pita (450 calories, 17 g fat)
- Guiltless Grilled Salmon (480 calories, 14 g fat)
- Guiltless Chicken Sandwich (490 calories, 8 g fat)
- Firecracker Tilapia (540 calories, 13 g fat)
- Guiltless Chicken Platter (580 calories, 9 g fat)
- Guiltless Black Bean Burger (650 calories, 12 g fat)
- Margarita Grilled Chicken (690 calories, 14 g fat)

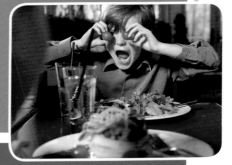

Friday's

- Key West Grouper (300 calories, 4 g fat)
- Dragonfire Chicken (437 calories, 8 g fat)
- Zen Chicken Pot Stickers (500 calories, 10 g fat)

Cracker Barrel

- Vegetable Soup with Westminster Crackers (115 calories, 2 g fat)
- Country Vegetable Plate: Sweet Whole Baby Carrots, Country Green Beans, Whole Kernel Corn, and Turnip Greens (380 calories, 20 g fat)
- Country Dinner Plate: Homemade Chicken n' Dumplings with Country Green Beans and Sweet Whole Baby Carrots (390 calories, 10 g fat)
- Country Dinner Plate: Grilled Chicken Tenders with Whole Kernel Corn and Country Green Beans (400 calories, 18 g fat)

Perkins

- BLT Chicken Breast Salad, no cheese, dressing on the side* (365 calories, 11 g fat)
- Chicken Noodle Soup with side salad and fat-free Italian dressing (365 calories, 10 g fat)
- Chicken Caesar Salad, dressing on the side* (410 calories, 17 g fat)

* Dressing not included in values shown.

Bob Evans

- Slow-Roasted Turkey (114 calories, 4 g fat)
- Potato-Crusted Flounder (254 calories, 17 g fat)
- Multigrain Hotcake* (322 calories, 10 g fat)
- Fruit & Yogurt Plate (403 calories, 2 g fat)
- Chicken Salad Plate (763 calories, 7 g fat)

* Ask if you can special order the multigrain hotcake batter mixed with blueberries. If not, top your hotcake with blueberries and omit the butter and syrup.

Mimi's Cafe

Dr. Colbert
Approved

- ½ Fresh Roasted Turkey Breast Sandwich (336 calories, 9 g fat)
- Old Fashioned Buckeye Oatmeal (426 calories, 2 g fat)
- Slow-Roasted Turkey Breast, no gravy, with jasmine rice and fresh steamed vegetables (541 calories, 15 g fat)
- Market Fish* with jasmine rice and fresh steamed vegetables (565 calories, 10 g fat)
- Chicken & Fruit Salad with nonfat French dressing (599 calories, 9 g fat)

* Average values provided. They may vary depending on the type of fish available.

Seasons 52

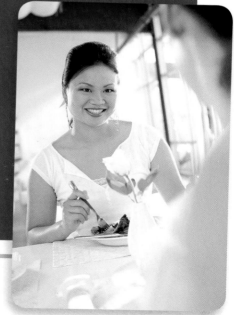

Seasons 52 is not yet a national chain, but I hope that it will be someday. I see it as a prototype of the restaurant of the future and could not pass up the opportunity to mention it as a restaurant I highly recommend. Foods are served at their peak of freshness and grilled over wood fires or oven roasted. Everything on the menu is 500 calories or less. Right now, there are only a few locations in Florida and Georgia. If you are lucky enough to be near one, I encourage you to patronize this excellent source of healthy dining.

TIPS FOR HEALTHY KIDS

GETTING KIDS TO EAT HEALTHILY

FOR THE FIRST TIME in two hundred years, children in America may have a shorter life expectancy than their parents. The reason? Obesity! A report in the *New England Journal of Medicine* predicts that the rise in childhood obesity could reduce the lifespan of this current generation of children by five years.[1] All parents know what a challenge it can be to get kids to enjoy healthy foods at times. But in light of the epidemic of childhood obesity we're facing, teaching kids to eat living foods is one of the most important things parents can do. On these pages you'll find tips and ideas that I hope will inspire you to start your child on a lifelong love of living foods.

Get Them Involved

One of the easiest ways to get your kids to try new foods is to get them involved in selecting food at the grocery store. Let your child be in charge of picking out one new fruit or vegetable a week. Teach them to read food labels, and make a game out of finding the healthiest bread, pasta, or cereal product. At home, make kids part of meal preparations by having them:

- Wash fruits and vegetables being prepared
- Tear up lettuce for salads
- Snap green beans
- Shuck corn on the cob
- Mash potatoes with a potato masher
- Break off broccoli and cauliflower florets
- Measure fruits and veggies for recipes
- Combine fruits in a bowl for fruit salad
- Use a mister to spray olive oil on salads or other foods during preparation

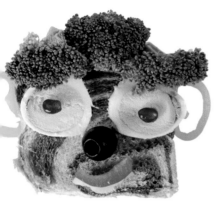

Get "Fresh"!

If cooked veggies turn your children off, don't fall into the trap of slathering them with butter or cheese to make them more palatable. Try serving raw carrots, snap peas, broccoli, and cauliflower. It's surprising how, once the mushy consistency from being cooked is gone, many people love the fresh version of the same vegetables they thought they hated.

Make It Fun

A trip down the cereal aisle at your grocery store will tell you that children are drawn in by colorful packaging. Use this to your advantage. Purchase some fun storage containers (look for bright colors or your child's favorite cartoon character) and store fruits, vegetables, whole-grain cereals, and snack bars in these containers. Put them on a special shelf at your child's eye level in the refrigerator or pantry. When your child asks you for a snack, let him pull out his "special snack" container and help himself.

Avoid Mealtime Battles

Mealtime can be a stressful battleground with young children. If this has been the case at your house, don't use this time to start adding healthy foods to your child's diet. Try working them in as snacks throughout the day. Associate eating these foods with things she enjoys doing, and she's much more likely to accept them.

Move It!

Healthy eating is not enough to conquer obesity; it must be accompanied by an active lifestyle. If you notice your child spending inordinate amounts of time on the couch or playing video or computer games, don't just tell him to go ride his bike—do it with him! Other activities kids and parents can do together:

- Walk the family pet
- Play catch with a softball or baseball
- Play some backyard volleyball, kickball, or badminton
- Take a picnic lunch to the park
- Join a local YMCA or health club with family-style fitness programs

NOTES

1—Living Food vs. Dead Food

1. *California Healthline*, "Life Expectancy Increases to 77.6 Years in U.S., Study Finds," December 9, 2005. *California Healthline* is published for the California HealthCare Foundation by the Advisory Board Company.

2. *Rural Migration News*, "How We Eat," vol. 3, no. 4, October 1996, http://migration.ucdavis .edu/rmn/more.php?id=158_0_5_0 (accessed September 5, 2008).

2—Your Body Is a Temple

1. Matthew Herper, "The Hidden Cost of Obesity," Forbes.com, November 24, 2006, http://www.forbes.com/business/2006/07/19/obesity-fat-costs_cx_mh_0720obesity.html (accessed September 5, 2008).

2. Roy Walford, *Beyond the 120-Year Diet* (New York: Four Walls Eight Windows, 2000), 45–49, referenced in K. C. Craichy, *Super Health* (Minneapolis, MN: Bronze Bow Publishing, 2005), 57.

3. C. C. Cowie et al., "Prevalence of Diabetes and Impaired Fasting Glucose in Adults in the U.S. Population: National Health and Nutrition Examination Survey (NHANES) 1999–2000," *Diabetes Care* 29, no. 6 (June 2006): 1263–1268.

4. Brian Wansink, PhD, *Mindless Eating: Why We Eat More Than We Think* (New York: Bantam, 2007), 140–145.

3—What the Bible Says About Food

1. G. E. Fraser and D. J. Shavlik, "Ten Years of Life: Is It a Matter of Choice?" *Archives of Internal Medicine* 161, no. 13 (2001): 1645–1652.

2. T. J. Key et al., "Mortality in Vegetarians and Non-Vegetarians: A Collaborative Analysis of 8300 Deaths Among 76,000 Men and Women in Five Prospective Studies," *Public Health Nutrition* 1, no. 1 (March 1998): 33–41.

3. Jeanie Lerche Davis, "America's Food Trends: People Eating Healthy, Eating at Home," WebMD Medical News, http://www.webmd .com/content/article/72/81891.htm (accessed September 8, 2008).

4—What to Avoid

1. Real Truth.org, "Eating Yourself to Death," July 8, 2004, http://www.realtruth.org/articles/244-eytd.html (accessed October 10, 2008).

2. FAO.org, "Country Profiles: United States of America," *FAO Statistical Yearbook*, http://www .fao.org/statistics/yearbook/vol_1_2/pdf/United -States-of-America.pdf (accessed September 5, 2008).

3. Helen Wright et al., *Foods Commonly Eaten in the United States* (Washington DC: USDA, 2002), http://www.ars.usda.gov/SP2UserFiles/Place/12355000/pdf/Portion.pdf (accessed September 5, 2008).

4. Gene Marine and Judith Van Allen, *Food Pollution—the Violation of Our Inner Ecology* (Canada: Holt, Rinehart, and Winston, 1972), referenced in Judy Campbell, BSc, et al., "Nutritional Characteristics of Organic, Freshly Stone-ground, Sourdough and Conventional Breads," http://www.eap.mcgill.ca/Publications/EAP35.htm (accessed September 8, 2008), referenced in Don Colbert, MD, "Curbing the Toxic Onslaught," *NutriNews*, August 2005.

5. Robert Preidt, "Pesticide Exposure Causes Damage to Nervous System, Brain," HealthDay News, August 4, 2006, http://www.refluxissues .com/ms/news/534119/main.html (accessed September 8, 2008).

6. Alberto Ascherio et al., "Pesticide Exposure and Risk of Parkinson's Disease," *Annals of Neurology* (July 2006): referenced in "Pesticide Exposure Associated With Incidence of Parkinson's Disease," press release from EurekAlert .com, June 26, 2006, http://www.eurekalert .org/pub_releases/2006-06/jws-pea061906.php (accessed September 8, 2008).

7. A. Blair et al., "Clues to Cancer Etiology From Studies of Farmers," *Scandinavian Journal of Work Environment, and Health* 18, no. 4 (1992): 209–215, referenced in Aaron Blair, PhD, "Risk Factors: Pesticides," National Cancer Institute, http://rex.nci.nih.gov/NCI_Pub_Interface/raterisk/risks99.html (accessed September 8, 2008).

8. *Idaho Observer,* "Bleaching Agent in Flour Linked to Diabetes," http://proliberty.com/observer/20050718.htm (accessed February 20, 2006), referenced in Colbert, "Curbing the Toxic Onslaught."

9. Pollution in People, "PCBs and DDT: Banned but Still with Us," July 2006, http://www.pollutioninpeople.org/toxics/pcbs_ddt (accessed September 8, 2008).

10. Thea Deley, "Food Dyes Linked to Hyper Kids, Group Asks FDA to Ban," InformifyNews.com, June 6, 2008, http://www.informify.com/top-stories/48-health/199-food-dyes-linked-to-hyper-kids-group-asks-fda-to-ban (accessed October 15, 2008). Also, Center for Science in the Public Interest, "CSPI Urges FDA to Ban Artificial Food Dyes Linked to Behavior Problems," http://www.cspinet.org/new/200806022.html (accessed October 15, 2008).

11. TruthinLabeling.org, "Collected Reports of Endocrine Disorders, Retinal Degeneration, and Adverse Reactions Caused by MSG," http://www.truthinlabeling.org/adversereactions.html (accessed September 8, 2008).

12. Medline Plus Encyclopedia, s.v. "Chinese Restaurant Syndrome," http://www.nlm.nih.gov/medlineplus/ency/article/001126.htm (accessed September 8, 2008).

13. Educate-Yourself.org, "Sugar," Nutrition, the Key to Energy, http://educate-yourself.org/nutrition/#sugar (accessed September 8, 2008).

14. Becky Hand, "The Hunt for Hidden Sugar: How Much of the Sweet Stuff Is Hiding Your Foods?" BabyFit.com, http://www.babyfit.com/articles.asp?id=685 (accessed September 8, 2008).

15. S. J. Schoenthaler and I. D. Bier, "The Effect of Vitamin-Mineral Supplementation on Juvenile Delinquency Among American Schoolchildren: A Randomized, Double-blind Placebo-controlled Trial," *Journal of Alternative and Complementary Medicine* 6, no. 1 (February 2000): 7–17.

16. Dani Veracity, "The Politics of Sugar: Why Your Government Lies to You About This Disease-Promoting Ingredient," NaturalNews .com, July 21, 2005, http://www.naturalnews.com/z009797.html (accessed September 8, 2008).

17. Gary Farr, "The Thymus Gland," Become HealthyNow.com, http://www.becomehealthynow.com/article/bodyimmune/961/3/ (accessed October 15, 2008).

18. Joseph Mercola, MD, "The Potential Dangers of Sucralose: Reader Testimonials," Mercola.com, http://www.mercola.com (accessed July 25, 2006).

19. Food and Diet, "Splenda," http://www.foodanddiet.com/NewFiles/splenda.html (accessed September 8, 2008).

20. Stephen Fox, "New Mexico Senate Bill to Ban Artificial Sweetener Aspartame as Neurotoxic Carcinogen," *NewswireToday* - /newswire/ - Santa Fe, New Mexico, January 17, 2006.

21. Federal Register of the U.S. Food and Drug Administration, Center for Food Safety and Applied Nutrition, "Food Additives Permitted for Direct Addition to Food for Human Consumption: Sucralose," vol. 63, no. 64, April 3, 1998, 16417–16443, http://www.cfsan.fda.gov/%7Elrd/fr980403.html (accessed September 8, 2008).

22. Daniel DeNoon, "Drink More Diet Soda, Gain More Weight?" WebMD Medical News, June 13, 2005, http://www.webmd.com/content/Article/107/108476.htm (accessed September 8, 2008).

23. Bonnie Liebman, "The Whole Grain Guide," *Nutrition Action HealthLetter,* March 1997, http://www.cspinet.org/nah/wwheat.html (accessed September 8, 2008).

24. Eric Schlosser, *Fast Food Nation* (New York: Houghton Mifflin, 2001).

25. Paul Appleby, "Do Vegetarians Live Longer?" lecture notes on a talk given to student members of the Oxford Green Party, Friends Meeting House, Oxford, UK, March 1, 2002, http://www.ivu.org/oxveg/Talks/veglongevity.html (accessed September 8, 2008); also, T. J. Key, G. K. Davey, and P. N. Appleby, "Health Benefits of a Vegetarian Diet," *Proceedings of the Nutrition Society* 58, no. 2 (May 1999): 271–275.

26. Cancer Prevention Coalition, "Hot Dogs and Nitrites," http://www.preventcancer.com/consumers/food/hotdogs.htm (accessed September 8, 2008).

27. Food Safety and Inspection Service, "Hot Dogs and Food Safety," U.S. Department of Agriculture, http://www.fsis.usda.gov/Fact_Sheets/Hot_Dogs/index.asp (accessed October 22, 2008).

28. Ibid.

29. "Nutritional Information from Bob Evans Menu," provided by the company Web site, http://www.bobevans.com (accessed September 8, 2008). The information provided was last updated September 8, 2008.

30. BanTransFats.com, "New Labeling," http://www.bantransfats.com/newlabeling.html (accessed September 8, 2008).

31. Stephanie Lingafelter, "Supersized Fat in America," Mother Earth Living, http://www.motherearthliving.com/issues/motherearthliving/whole_foods/Trans-Fat-Risks_227-1.html (accessed September 8, 2008).

32. American Heart Association, "Limiting Fats and Cholesterol," American Heart Association, http://www.americanheart.org/presenter.jhtml?identifier=323 (accessed September 8, 2008).

33. Calorie King, "Calories and Carbs in Fats: Animal Fats or Lards, Meat Drippings," http://www.calorieking.com/foods/food/carbs-calories-in-fats-animal-fats-or-lards-meat-drippings_Y2lkPTMzNDIxJmJpZDoxJmZpZD02ODA1NSZlaWQ9Mzc1MDIyNTQmcG9zPTgmcGFyPSZrZXk9YmFjb24.html (accessed September 8, 2008).

5—Stayin' Alive With Living Foods

1. American Chemical Society, "Research at Great Lakes Meeting Shows More Vitamin C in Organic Oranges Than Conventional Oranges," June 2, 2002 press release, http://www.sciencedaily.com/releases/2002/06/020603071017.htm (accessed September 8, 2008).

2. R. Hites, et al., "Farm-Raised Salmon Contain More Toxins Than Wild Salmon," Science, January 9, 2004, http://www.breastcancer.org/research_farm_raised_salmon.html (accessed February 20, 2006).

3. Environmental Working Group, "Summary—PCBs in Farmed Salmon," July 2003, http://www.ewg.org/reports/farmedPCBs (accessed September 8, 2008).

4. ConsumerReports.org, "When Buying Organic Pays (and Doesn't)," June 2, 2008, http://blogs.consumerreports.org/baby/2008/06/organic-food.html?resultPageIndex=1&resultIndex=1&searchTerm=buying%20organic (accessed September 8, 2008).

5. U.S. Department of Health and Human Services, and U.S. Department of Agriculture, Dietary Guidelines for Americans 2005, http://healthierus.gov/dietaryguidelines (accessed September 8, 2008).

6. Life Extension Journal, "Vegetables Without Vitamins," March 2001, http://www.lef.org/magazine/mag2001/mar2001_report_vegetables.html (accessed September 8, 2008).

7. Carole Davis and Etta Saltos, Recommendations Over Time (Washington DC: USDA/ERS, n.d.), 33, http://www.ers.usda.gov/publications/aib750/aib750b.pdf (accessed September 3, 2008).

8. BestDietTips.com, "Glycemic Index List of Foods," http://www.bestdiettips.com/html/glycemic_index.php (accessed September 8, 2008).

9. Pew Initiative on Food and Biotechnology, "Genetically Modified Crops in the United States," http://www.pewtrusts.org/news_room_detail.aspx?id=17950 (accessed October 15, 2008).

10. Whole Grain Council, "Easy Ways to Enjoy Whole Grains," http://www.wholegrainscouncil.org/whole-grains-101/easy-ways-to-enjoy-whole-grains (accessed September 8, 2008).

11. NorthwesterNutrition, "Nutrition Fact Sheet: Dietary Fiber," Northwestern University, http://www.feinberg.northwestern.edu/nutrition/factsheets/fiber.html (accessed September 8, 2008).

12. Ibid.

13. Ibid.

14. Ibid.

15. T. A. Mori and L. J. Beilin, "Omega-3 Fatty Acids and Inflammation," Current Atherosclerosis Report 6, no. 6 (November 2004): 461–467; W. E. Hardman, "n-3 Fatty Acids and Cancer Therapy," Journal of Nutrition. 134, suppl. 12 (December 2004): 3427S–3430S; A. A. Berbert et al., "Supplementation of Fish Oil and Olive Oil in

Patients With Rheumatoid Arthritis," *Nutrition* 21, no. 2 (February 2005): 131–136; P. Guesnet et al., "Analysis of the 2nd Symposium: Anomalies of Fatty Acids, Ageing and Degenerating Pathologies," *Reproduction Nutrition Development* 44, no. 3 (May–June 2004): 263–271; J. A. Conquer et al., "Fatty Acid Analysis of Blood Plasma of Patients With Alzheimer's D, Other Types of Dementia, and Cognitive Impairment," *Lipids* 35, no. 12 (December 2000): 1305–1312; L. A. Horrocks and Y. K. Yeo, "Health Benefits of Docosahexaenoic Acid (DHA)," *Pharmacological Research* 40, no. 3 (September 1999): 211–225; E. M. Hjerkinn et al., "Influence of Long-Term Intervention With Dietary Counseling, Long-Chain n-3 Fatty Acid Supplements, or Both on Circulating Markers of Endothelial Activation in Men With Long-Standing Hyperlipidemia," *Alternative Medicine Review* 81, no. 3 (March 2005): 583–589; and J. A. Nettleton and R. Katz, "n-3 Long-Chain Polyunsaturated Fatty Acids in Type 2 Diabetes: A Review," *Journal of the American Dietetic Association* 105, no. 3 (March 2005): 428–440.

16. M. G. Enig, *Trans Fatty Acids in the Food Supply: A Comprehensive Report Covering 60 Years of Research*, 2nd edition (Silver Spring, MD: Enig Associates, Inc., 1995).

17. Don Colbert, MD, *What Would Jesus Eat?* (Nashville, TN: Thomas Nelson, 2001).

18. Essence-of-Life.com, compiled from "Alkaline/Acidic Food Charts," http://www.essense-of-life.com/moreinfo/foodcharts.htm (accessed September 8, 2008).

19. George Mateljan Foundation, "What Is the Special Nutritional Power Found in Fruits and Vegetables?" http://www.whfoods.com/genpage.php?tname=faq&dbid=4 (accessed September 8, 2008).

20. Tiesha D. Johnson, BSN, RN, "All About Supplements: Blueberries," *Life Extension*, September 2006, 88.

21. Ibid.

22. Judy McBride, "High-ORAC Foods May Slow Aging," U.S. Department of Agriculture, Agricultural Research Service, February 8, 1999, http://www.ars.usda.gov/is/pr/1999/990208.htm

(accessed September 8, 2008).

23. E. Giovannucci et al., "Intake of Carotenoids and Retinol in Relation to Risk of Prostate Cancer," *Journal of the National Cancer Institute* 87 (December 6, 1995): 1767–1776.

24. *Bolton Evening News*, "Carrots Cut Cancer Risk," February 9, 2005, abstract accessed at http://archive.thisislancashire.co.uk/2005/02/09/445271.html (accessed September 8, 2008).

25. J. M. Seddon et al., "Dietary Carotenoids, Vitamins A, C, and E, and Advanced Age-Related Macular Degeneration," *Journal of the American Medical Association* 272 (1994): 1413–1420.

26. Harvard School of Public Health, "Fruits and Vegetables," http://www.hsph.harvard.edu/nutritionsource/fruits.html (accessed September 8, 2008).

27. Alexander Schauss et al., "Antioxidant Capacity and Other Bioactivities of the Freeze-Dried Amazonian Palm Berry, Euterpe Oleraceae Mart. (Acai)," *Journal of Agriculture and Food Chemistry* 54, no. 22 (November 1, 2006), http://pubs.acs.org/cgi-bin/abstract.cgi/jafcau/2006/54/i22/abs/jf060976g.html (accessed October 16, 2008).

28. Marc Kusinitz, "Cancer Protection Compound Abundant in Broccoli Sprouts," September 15, 1997, Johns Hopkins, http://www.hopkinsmedicine.org/press/1997/SEPT/970903.HTM (accessed September 10, 2008).

29. Tiesha D. Johnson, BSN, RN, "Powerful Protection for Aging Arteries—and Much More," *LE Magazine*, May 2007, http://search.lef.org/LEFCMS/aspx/PrintVersionMagic.aspx?CmsID=114814 (accessed October 5, 2008).

6—Targeting Your Intake of Specific Antioxidants, Vitamins, and Minerals

1. X. Wu et al., "Lipophilic and Hydrophilic Antioxidant Capacities of Common Foods in the United States," *Journal of Agricultural and Food Chemistry* 52, no. 12 (June 9, 2004): 4026–4037.

2. Alanna Moshfegh, Joseph Goodman, and Linda Cleveland, "What We Eat in America,

NHANES 2001–2002: Usual Nutrient Intakes From Food Compared to Dietary Reference Intakes," U.S. Department of Agriculture, Agricultural Research Service, http://www.ars.usda.gov/research/publications/publications.htm?SEQ_NO_115=184176 (accessed September 9, 2008).

3. National Institutes of Health Office of Dietary Supplements, "Dietary Supplement Fact Sheet: Vitamin A and Carotenoids," NIH Clinical Center, http://ods.od.nih.gov/factsheets/vitamina.asp (accessed September 9, 2008).

4. Ibid.

5. P. Mecocci et al., "Plasma Antioxidants and Longevity: A Study on Healthy Centenarians," *Free Radical Biology and Medicine* 28, no. 8 (September 2000): 1243–1248.

6. Joseph E. Pizzorno Jr. and Michael T. Murray, eds., *Textbook of Natural Medicine* (New York: Churchill Livingston, 1999), 1007–1013.

7. National Institutes of Health Office of Dietary Supplements, "Dietary Supplement Fact Sheet: Vitamin A and Carotenoids."

8. K. J. Rothman, L. L. Moore, and M. R. Singer, "Tertogenecity of High Vitamin A Intake," *New England Journal of Medicine* 333 (1995): 1369–1373.

9. Pizzorno and Murray, *Textbook of Natural Medicine*, 1013.

10. From an e-mail from Cathy Leet, BSN, Director of Market Development, Integrative Therapeutics Inc., to author's office, Tuesday, January 31, 2006.

11. Moshfegh, Goodman, and Cleveland, "What We Eat in America, NHANES 2001–2002."

12. J. E. Leklem, "Vitamin B$_6$," in M. E. Shils et al., ed., *Modern Nutrition in Health and Disease*, 9th ed. (Baltimore: Williams and Wilkins, 1999), 413–421.

13. National Institutes of Health Office of Dietary Supplements, "Dietary Supplement Fact Sheet: Vitamin B$_6$," NIH Clinical Center, http://ods.od.nih.gov/factsheets/vitaminb6.asp (accessed September 9, 2008); and George Mateljan Foundation, "Vitamin B$_6$," World's Healthiest Foods, http://www.whfoods.com/genpage.php?tname=nutrient&dbid=108#foodsources (accessed September 9, 2008).

14. WrongDiagnosis.com, "Symptoms of Pyridoxine Deficiency," http://www.wrongdiagnosis.com/p/pyridoxine_deficiency/symptoms.htm (accessed October 5, 2008).

15. National Institutes of Health Office of Dietary Supplements, "Dietary Supplement Fact Sheet: Vitamin B$_6$"; and "Vitamin B$_6$."

16. Moshfegh, Goodman, and Cleveland, "What We Eat in America, NHANES 2001–2002."

17. Ohio State University, "Extension Fact Sheet: Vitamin C (Ascorbic Acid)," http://ohioline.osu.edu/hyg-fact/5000/5552.html (accessed September 9, 2008).

18. Lester Packer, PhD, *The Antioxidant Miracle* (New York: John Wiley and Sons, Inc., 1999).

19. WrongDiagnosis.com, "Symptoms of Vitamin C Deficiency," http://www.wrongdiagnosis.com/v/vitamin_c_deficiency/symptoms.htm (accessed September 9, 2008).

20. Pizzorno and Murray, *Textbook of Natural Medicine*, 549, 836, 915–916.

21. Shands Health Care, "Vitamin C," in the Illustrated Health Encyclopedia, http://www.shands.org/health/Health%20Illustrated%20Encyclopedia/1/002404.htm (accessed October 5, 2008).

22. Janet Raloff, "Understanding Vitamin D Deficiency," *Science News Online*, http://www.sciencenews.org/view/generic/id/6123/title/Food_for_Thought__Understanding_Vitamin_D_Deficiency (accessed September 9, 2008).

23. Phyllis A. Balch, CNC, *Prescription for Nutritional Healing*, rev. and expanded edition (New York: Avery Books, 2000), 21.

24. National Institutes of Health Office of Dietary Supplements, "Dietary Supplement Fact Sheet: Vitamin D," NIH Clinical Center, http://ods.od.nih.gov/factsheets/vitamind.asp (accessed September 9, 2008).

25. Ibid.

26. Ibid.

27. National Osteoporosis Foundation, "Prevention: Calcium and Vitamin D," http://www.nof.org/prevention/calcium2.htm (accessed September 9, 2008).

28. According to an analysis published in 2004 and based on the Third National Health and Nutrition Examination Survey (NHANES III).

29. National Institutes of Health Office of

Dietary Supplements, "Dietary Supplement Fact Sheet: Vitamin D."

30. Ibid.

31. Kirk Fernandes and Joseph Brownstein, "Pediatricians Double Vitamin D Requirement," October 13, 2008, http://abcnews.go.com/Health/story?id=6006566&page=1 (accessed October 17, 2008).

32. Moshfegh, Goodman, and Cleveland, "What We Eat in America, NHANES 2001–2002."

33. Ohio State University, "Extension Fact Sheet: Vitamin E," http://ohioline.osu.edu/hyg-fact/5000/5554.html (accessed September 9, 2008).

34. K. J. Helzlsouer et al., "Association Between Alpha-Tocopherol, Gamma-Tocopherol, Selenium, and Subsequent Prostate Cancer," *Journal of the National Cancer Institute* 92, no. 24 (December 2000): 1966–1967.

35. National Institutes of Health Office of Dietary Supplements, "Dietary Supplement Fact Sheet: Vitamin E," NIH Clinical Center, http://ods.od.nih.gov/factsheets/vitamine.asp (accessed September 9, 2008).

36. Ibid.

37. Eva Lonn, MD, MSc, et al., "Effects of Long-Term Vitamin E Supplementation on Cardiovascular Events and Cancer," *Journal of the American Medical Association* 293, no. 11 (March 16, 2005): 1338–1347.

38. Moshfegh, Goodman, and Cleveland, "What We Eat in America, NHANES 2001–2002."

39. NorthwesterNutrition, "Nutrition Fact Sheet: Vitamin K," Northwestern University, http://www.feinberg.northwestern.edu/nutrition/factsheets/vitamin-k.html (accessed September 9, 2008).

40. Ibid.

41. J. M. Geleijnse et al., "Dietary Intake of Menaquinone Is Associated With a Reduced Risk of Coronary Heart Disease: The Rotterdam Study," *Journal of Nutrition* 134, no. 11 (November 2004): 3100–3105, referenced in William Davis, MD, "Protecting Bone and Arterial Health

With Vitamin K2," *Life Extension Magazine*, March 2008, http://www.lef.org/magazine/mag2008/mar2008_Protecting-Bone-And-Arterial-Health-With-Vitamin-K2_01.htm (accessed October 17, 2008).

42. A. M. Stapleton and R. L. Rydall, "Crystal Matrix Protein—Getting Blood Out of a Stone," *Mineral and Electrolyte Metabolism* 20, no. 6 (1994): 399–409.

43. Balch, *Prescription for Nutritional Healing*, 23.

44. Moshfegh, Goodman, and Cleveland, "What We Eat in America, NHANES 2001–2002."

45. National Institutes of Health Office of Dietary Supplements, "Dietary Supplement Fact Sheet: Magnesium," NIH Clinical Center, http://ods.od.nih.gov/factsheets/magnesium.asp (accessed September 9, 2008).

46. National Institutes of Health Office of Dietary Supplements, "Dietary Supplement Fact Sheet: Calcium," NIH Clinical Center, http://ods.od.nih.gov/factsheets/calcium.asp (accessed September 9, 2008).

47. Ibid.

48. Ibid.

49. CalciumInfo.com, "Important News on Osteoporosis and Bone Health," http://www.calciuminfo.com/, referencing *Bone Health and Osteoporosis: A Report of the Surgeon General*, available at http://www.surgeongeneral.gov/topics/bonehealth/ (accessed September 9, 2008).

50. Moshfegh, Goodman, and Cleveland, "What We Eat in America, NHANES 2001–2002."

51. University of Maryland Medical Center, "Potassium," fact sheet, http://www.umm.edu/altmed/ConsSupplements/Potassiumcs.html (accessed September 9, 2008).

52. Hopkins Technology, LLC, "Food Sources of Potassium," http://www.hoptechno.com/bookfoodsourceK.htm (accessed September 9, 2008).

7—What to Eat With Caution

1. PublicCitizen.org, "Is Irradiated Food Safe?" http://www.citizen.org/print_article.cfm?ID=1423 (accessed September 9, 2008).

2. J. D. Decuypere, MD, "Radiation, Irradiation and Our Food Supply," The Decuypere Report, http://www.healthalternatives2000.com/food_supply_report.html (accessed September 9, 2008).

3. PublicCitizen.org, "Is Irradiated Food Safe?"

4. Decuypere, "Radiation, Irradiation and Our Food Supply."

5. University of Michigan Integrative Medicine, "Healthy Fats," http://www.med.umich.edu/umim/clinical/pyramid/fats.htm (accessed September 9, 2008).

6. C. A. Daley et al., "A Literature Review of the Value-Added Nutrients Found in Grass-fed Beef Products," California State University–Chico, draft manuscript, June 2005, http://www.csuchico.edu/agr/grassfedbeef/health-benefits/index.html (accessed September 9, 2008).

7. Associated Press, "Red Meat Raises Breast Cancer Risk," MSNBC.com, February 7, 2007, http://www.msnbc.msn.com/id/15702642/print/1/displaymode/1098/ (accessed October 17, 2008).

8. James Buchanan Brady Urological Institute, "Racemase: A New Marker for Cancer, and More," Prostate Cancer Update, Winter 2003, http://urology.jhu.edu/newsletter/prostate_cancer67.php (accessed October 17, 2008).

9. Emily Oken, MD, et al., "Decline in Fish Consumption Among Pregnant Women After a National Mercury Advisory," Obstetrics and Gynecology 102 (2003): 346–351, http://www.greenjournal.org/cgi/content/full/102/2/346 (accessed September 9, 2008).

10. Lynn R. Goldman, MD, MPH, et al., "American Academy of Pediatrics: Technical Report: Mercury in the Environment: Implications for Pediatricians," Pediatrics 108, no. 1 (July 2001): 197–205.

11. Educate-Yourself.org, "Dairy Products," Nutrition, the Key to Energy, http://www.educate-yourself.org/nutrition/#dairyproducts (accessed September 9, 2008).

12. George Mateljan Foundation, "Pasteurization," http://www.whfoods.com/genpage.php?tname=george&dbid=149#answer

13. USDA, "The Dangers of Raw Milk," Food-Facts, October 2006. Also, Cornell University, "Why Pasteurize? The Dangers of Consuming Raw Milk," Dairy Science Facts, 1998.

14. L. Maia and A. deMendonca, "Does Caffeine Intake Protect From Alzheimer's Disease?" European Journal of Neurology 9, no. 4 (July 2002): 377–382.

15. Eduardo Salazar-Martinez, MD, et al., "Coffee Consumption and Risk for Type 2 Diabetes Mellitus," Annals of Internal Medicine 140 (January 6, 2004), 1–8.

16. Susan Yara, "Coffee Perks, Forbes Online, October 12, 2005, http://www.forbes.com/health/2005/10/11/coffee-health-benefits-cx_sy_1012feat_ls.html (accessed September 9, 2008).

17. Marc Leduc, "Is Coffee Good or Bad for Your Health," Healing Daily Web site, http://www.healingdaily.com/detoxification-diet/coffee.htm (accessed September 9, 2008).

18. General Conference Nutrition Council, "A Position Statement on the Use of Caffeine," http://www.nadadventist.org/hm/gcnc/caffeine/caffeine.htm (accessed September 9, 2008).

19. White Tea Central, "White Tea vs. Green Tea," http://www.whiteteacentral.com/white-teavsgreen.html (accessed October 17, 2008).

20. Mark Jeantheau, "Styrofoam Cups—Clouds in Your Coffee?" Grinning Planet, November 1, 2005, http://www.grinningplanet.com/2005/11-01/styrofoam-cups-article.htm (accessed September 9, 2008).

21. I-Min Lee and Ralph S. Paffenbarger Jr., "Life Is Sweet: Candy Consumption and Longevity," British Medical Journal 317 (December 19, 1998): 1683–1684.

22. University of Alabama–Birmingham Health System, "Chocolate Works Against Hypertension," http://www.health.uab.edu/show.asp?durki=84606 (accessed February 22, 2006).

8—What to Drink

1. Environmental Protection Agency, "Where Does My Drinking Water Come From?" Drinking Water, http://www.epa.gov/region7/kids/drnk_b.htm (accessed September 9, 2008).

2. Wellness Filter, "The Forgotten Secret of Health: Are You Missing the Most Important

Ingredient for Optimum Health?" http://www
.wellnessfilter.com/about/TheForgottenSecret
ofHealth.pdf (accessed September 9, 2008).

3. Barbara Levine, RD, PhD, "Hydration 101:
The Case for Drinking Enough Water," Health
and Nutrition News, http://www.myhealt
hpointe.com/health_Nutrition_news/index
.cfm?Health=10 (accessed September 9, 2008).

4. Tammy Darling, "Water Works," *Vibrant Life*,
January 2001, http://www.findarticles
.com/p/articles/mi_m0826/is_1_17/ai_
69371786 (accessed September 9, 2008).

5. Levine, "Hydration 101: The Case for
Drinking Enough Water."

6. Lori Ferme, "Water, Water Everywhere:
How Much Should You Drink?" American
Dietetic Association, http://www.eatright.org/
cps/rde/xchg/ada/hs.xsl/media_3173_ENU_
HTML.htm (accessed September 9, 2008).

7. D. A. Mansfield, "What Percentage of the
Human Body Is Water, and How Is This Deter-
mined?" *Boston Globe*, http://www.boston.com/
globe/search/stories/health/how_and_why/
011298.htm (accessed January 30, 2006).

8. Ion Health, "How Much Water Should
You Drink," http://www.ionhealth.ca/id70.html
(accessed September 9, 2008). Also, Health4
youonline.com, "Dehydration—the Benefits of
Drinking Water," http://www.health4yo
uonline.com/article_dehydration.htm (accessed
September 9, 2008).

9. Beverage Marketing Corporation, "Bottled
Water Continues As Number 2 in 2004,"
International Bottled Water Association, http://
www.bottledwater.org/public/Stats_2004.doc
(accessed September 9, 2008).

10. Ibid.

11. NSF International, "Bottled Water Fact
Kit: Five Facts to Know About Bottled Water,"
http://www.nsf.org/consumer/newsroom/pdf/
fact_water_five.pdf (accessed September 9,
2008).

12. Natural Resources Defense Council,
"Bottled Water: Pure Drink or Pure Hype?"
http://www.nrdc.org/water/drinking/bw/exesum
.asp (accessed September 9, 2008).

13. Ibid.

14. Ibid.

15. NSF International, "Bottled Water Fact
Kit: Five Facts to Know About Bottled Water."

16. John Stossel, "Is Bottled Water Than
Tap?" ABC News, May 6, 2005, accessed
via http://abcnews.go.com/2020/Health/
story?id=728070&page=1 (accessed September
9, 2008).

17. Natural Resources Defense Council,
"Bottled Water: Pure Drink or Pure Hype?"

18. Ion Life, Inc., "Apples with Apples: How to
Choose a Water Filter System," http://www
.ionizers.org/water-filters.html (accessed
September 9, 2008); and Denise Moffat, MD,
"The Basics of Water," http://www.naturalh
ealthtechniques.com/BasicsofHealth/Water_
files/water_basics1.htm (accessed September 9,
2008).

19. Moffatt, "The Basics of Water."

20. Ion Life, Inc., "Apples with Apples: How
to Choose a Water Filter System" and Moffatt,
"The Basics of Water."

21. Ion Life, Inc., "Apples with Apples: How to
Choose a Water Filter System."

9—Shopping Tips

1. Rich Pirog, "How Far Do Your Fruit and
Vegetables Travel?" Leopold Center for Sustain-
able Agriculture, http://www.leopold.iastate
.edu/pubs/staff/ppp/food_chart0402.pdf
(accessed April 14, 2008).

2. AMA Annual Meeting Resolution 508
Antimicrobial Use and Resistance, June 2001,
referenced in Horizon Organic, "What Is
Organic?" http://www.horizonorganic.com/
health/whatis.html (accessed September 9,
2008).

3. Educate-Yourself.org, "Dairy Products."

4. Lisa Stark, "Sugary Treats or Cereal
Offenders?" ABCNews.com, October 1, 2008,
http://www.abcnews.go.com/print?id=5930710
(accessed October 17, 2008).

5. David Zinczenko and Matt Goulding,
Eat This Not That (New York: Rodale, 2008),
230–231.

6. U.S. Department of Health and Human Services, "Portion Distortion," National Institutes of Health, http://hp2010.nhlbihin.net/portion/ (accessed September 11, 2008).

7. Ed and Elisa McClure, *Eat Your Way to a Healthy Life* (Boerne, TX: Passport Life Center), 92. Ed and Elisa are founds of Passport Life Center. Used by permission.

8. Gail Burton, *The Candida Control Cookbook* (Fairfield, CT: Aslan Publishing, 1995), 40.

9. Ibid., 37.

10. McClure, *Eat Your Way to a Heal-thy Life*.

11. Karen Tripp in Chyrel's Kitchen, as viewed at http://www.linkline.com/personal/gingen/season/chilifre.htm.

12. McClure, *Eat Your Way to a Heal-thy Life*.

13. Ed McClure, *Eat Your Way to a Healthy Life* (Lake Mary, FL: Siloam, 2006), 188.

10—Dinner's Ready!—How to Store, Prepare, and Serve Food

1. Karen Karaszkiewicz, "Storing Food Too Long Cuts Nutrients," *Daily Collegian Online*, April 5, 2005, http://www.collegian.psu.edu/archive/2005/04/04-05-05tdc/04-05-05dscihealth-04.asp (accessed September 9, 2008).

2. Ibid.

3. Utah State Extension Service, "Nutri Q & A Chima: Food Storage and Nutrients," http://www.cindachima.com/Nonfiction/text/Food%20storage%20article%208-05.pdf (accessed September 9, 2008).

4. Healthy Alternatives, "What Are Enzymes?" Healthy Reflections: The Function of Enzymes in Nutrition, http://www.healthyalternativesinc.com/enzymes.htm (accessed September 9, 2008).

5. Good Eats Fan Page, "Cooking Oil Smoke Points," http://www.goodeatsfanpage.com/CollectedInfo/OilSmokePoints.htm (accessed October 5, 2008).

6. Janet Raloff, "Microwaves Bedevil a B Vitamin—Research Indicates Overcooking and Microwaving Meat and Dairy Foods Inactivate Vitamin B_{12}—Brief Article," *Science News* 153, February 14, 1998, http://www.findarticles.com/p/articles/mi_m1200/is_n7_v153/ai_20346932 (accessed September 9, 2008).

7. B. H. Blanc and H. U. Hertel, "Comparative Study of Food Prepared Conventionally and in the Microwave Oven," published by Raum & Zelt, 1992, in *Journal of the Science of Food and Agriculture* 3, no. 2 (2003): 43.

8. National Center on Addiction and Substance Abuse, "Casa and TV Land/Nick at Nite Report Shows Frequent Family Dinners Cut Teens' Substance Abuse Risk in Half," press release, September 13, 2005, http://www.casacolumbia.org/absolutenm/templates/PressReleases.aspx?articleid=405&zoneid=64 (accessed September 9, 2008).

11—On the Go?—Smart Choices for Dining Out

1. U.S. Food and Drug Administration, "Appendix A: Definitions of Nutrient Content Claims," *A Food Labeling Guide*, http://www.cfsan.fda.gov/~dms/2lg-xa.html (accessed September 22, 2008).

12—Tips for Healthy Kids

1. Pam Belluck, "Children's Life Expectancy Being Cut Short by Obesity," *New York Times*, March 17, 2005, http://www.nytimes.com/2005/03/17/health/17obese.html (accessed September 9, 2008).

A Personal Note

From Don Colbert

God desires to heal you of disease. His Word is full of promises that confirm His love for you and His desire to give you His abundant life. His desire includes more than physical health for you; He wants to make you whole in your mind and spirit as well through a personal relationship with His Son, Jesus Christ.

If you haven't met my best friend, Jesus, I would like to take this opportunity to introduce Him to you. It is very simple. If you are ready to let Him come into your life and become your best friend, all you need to do is sincerely pray this prayer:

Lord Jesus, I want to know You as my Savior and Lord. I believe You are the Son of God and that You died for my sins. I also believe You were raised from the dead and now sit at the right hand of the Father praying for me. I ask You to forgive me for my sins and change my heart so that I can be Your child and live with You eternally. Thank You for Your peace. Help me to walk with You so that I can begin to know You as my best friend and my Lord. Amen.

If you have prayed this prayer, you have just made the most important decision of your life. I rejoice with you in your decision and your new relationship with Jesus. Please contact my publisher at pray4me@strang.com so that we can send you some materials that will help you become established in your relationship with the Lord. We look forward to hearing from you.

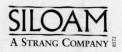